T0251635

Routledge Revivals

Exploration into Child Care

Originally published in 1971, this title explores childcare in the period between the Children Act of 1948 and the Seebohm Report of 1968. During this time Children's Departments and social work expanded beyond all expectations. In the developments of these two decades the author studies the history of the Child Care Service and a key example of the processes of social policy. The contents are a chronicle of events that shaped developments in the service in England and Wales during that time. Today it can be read and enjoyed in its historical context.

Exploration into Child Care

Peter Boss

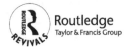

Routledge
Taylor & Francis Group

First published in 1971
by Routledge & Kegan Paul Ltd

This edition first published in 2023 by Routledge
4 Park Square, Milton Park, Abingdon, Oxon, OX14 4RN

and by Routledge
605 Third Avenue, New York, NY 10017

Routledge is an imprint of the Taylor & Francis Group, an informa business

© 1971 Peter Boss

Publisher's Note
The publisher has gone to great lengths to ensure the quality of this reprint but points out that some imperfections in the original copies may be apparent.

Disclaimer
The publisher has made every effort to trace copyright holders and welcomes correspondence from those they have been unable to contact.

A Library of Congress record exists under ISBN: 0710069650

ISBN: 978-1-032-44147-4 (hbk)
ISBN: 978-1-003-37075-8 (ebk)
ISBN: 978-1-032-44157-3 (pbk)

Book DOI 10.4324/9781003370758

Exploration into child care

by Peter Boss
University of Leicester,
School of Social Work

LONDON
ROUTLEDGE & KEGAN PAUL

First published 1971
by Routledge & Kegan Paul Ltd.,
Broadway House,
68-74 Carter Lane,
London, EC4V 5EL
Printed in Great Britain by
Northumberland Press Ltd.,
Gateshead 8
© Peter Boss 1971

ISBN 0 7100 6965 0

Contents

General editor's introduction

In its modern form, the Child Care service started from the publication of the Curtis Report and the enactment of the Children Act of 1948. It was envisaged then as a comparatively minor service for neglected and deprived children, headed by a local authority officer, probably a social worker, who could stand in loco parentis to them. In the next twenty years, both Children's Departments and social work were to expand beyond all expectations. The acquisition of preventive powers by Children's Departments under the 1963 Children and Young Persons Act, and the merging of two systems of residential care under the 1969 Act, have widened the scope of the work of Children's Departments. Instead of providing a small, specialized service, they are now providing in many areas a broad, family-based service with a number of developing specialisms. In the same period, social work has changed. Case-work techniques have become more sophisticated, and have been matched by a developing interest in group-work and community work.

The Seebohm Report of 1968, with its emphasis on area planning, unification of responsibility at the local level, and citizen participation, gives a new twist to the kaleidoscope. As Mr Boss says, the period between Curtis and Seebohm provides a distinctive period for study. In the developments of these two decades, we can study not only the history of the Child Care Service, but a key example of the processes of social policy. When we come to ask how a particular social problem is defined, what forces lead to the initiation of reform, how reform becomes law, and what consequences flow from new legal enactment, it is in studies of this kind that many of the answers can be found.

KATHLEEN JONES

1

Introduction

On 5 July 1948 the Children Act 1948 came into operation. It created the new child care service; at local level this took the form of establishing children's committees and departments; at central level it meant giving the Home Secretary general supervisory powers over the new service, setting up a child care inspectorate and an Advisory Council.

At the time the new service was hailed as a Children's Charter, offering a new deal for those children who had previously been in the care of public assistance and other local authority departments. The Curtis Committee, on whose report the Children Act was based, had expressed its view quite clearly that in future only one local authority committee should have responsibility for the care of children deprived of a normal home life and only one service should be devoted to meeting the needs of such children.

The Curtis Report of 1946 was something of a watershed in the history of the care of deprived children. The earlier period had been dominated by the Poor Law, but the Poor Law finally came to an end with the post-war programme of social reconstruction of which the Children Act formed a part.

The Act did not only give effect to the very necessary

reorganization of fragmented child care services, certainly, the Act laid down an administrative framework for action and defined the functions to be exercised, often in a quite detailed form, but it also gave expression to a new set of attitudes to be adopted towards the deprived child, different from those which characterized Poor Law policy. The new attitudes were intended to compensate the child for the effects of deprivation by providing him with the right kind of physical and emotional environment in which he could develop his natural potential.

At the outset the newly formed children's departments saw their work essentially in terms of care functions. The child was the focus of their activities. Sometimes they were led astray by the whims of fashion in methods of care, for instance, in a somewhat indiscriminate use of boarding out and family-group homes, but at least they followed the fashion in good faith. They had to be guided by their own experience for there was little evidence to help them see where they might be going wrong.

They were soon overwhelmed by the tide of children who were brought to public notice, they were understaffed and had to battle for scarce resources. Nonetheless, children's committees and their staffs put the service on its feet; and increasingly they acquired new functions. In 1958 they were empowered to act as adoption agencies, in 1959, under the Mental Health Act, they were given powers to accommodate mentally disordered children in residential establishments. Under the Matrimonial Proceedings Acts of 1958 and 1960 they were given the duty of acting as supervisors or fit persons to children entrusted to their care by the magistrates courts and the divorce courts. In 1963, the Children and Young Persons Act placed a duty on them to undertake preventive work with families so as to avoid children having to be received into care or coming before the courts. The most recent legislation, the Children and Young Persons Act 1969, conferred extensive functions on them in relation to young offenders.

The child care service was originally designed to meet the needs of a defined group of children but it has gradually shifted its orientation in the direction of the kind of family service foreshadowed in the Seebohm Report of 1968. The Seebohm Committee recommended the merging of child care with other personal social services to form a combined service which could meet the needs of whole families better than could a number of fragmented services. Implementation of the Seebohm proposals would spell the end of a separate child care service.

This book has been written as a result of the idea that the span between the Curtis and Seebohm reports provided a distinctive period for study. The contents therefore are a chronicle of events that have shaped developments in the service in England and Wales during this period.

2
The Children Act 1948

'Whose Children?'

Services for deprived children in the immediate post-war years were in administrative disarray. Responsibility for children who had come to public notice because of their family circumstances was divided up among a number of local and central government departments. Voluntary societies, too, continued to have a sizeable share of the work. The largest single group of children in public care was that under the official heading of 'destitute'. These were the children in the care of the local authorities' public assistance committees, ostensibly as 'poor persons in need of relief'. The governing statute was the Poor Law Act 1930, the latest in a long series of enactments for the relief of poor persons which reached back into the sixteenth century. Children in care under the 1930 legislation were those who had been orphaned or deserted or whose parents were physically or mentally ill, or for other reasons unable, or unwilling to look after them. Other children in public care were those who had come before the juvenile court, either as offenders or because they had been considered as being in need of care or protection, and who had been committed to the care of the local authority or sent to treatment institutions such as approved schools,

4

remand homes and probation hostels. In care, too, were mentally disordered and defective children, handicapped children who were being educated away from home, war-orphaned and evacuated children who had not returned to their homes at the end of hostilities. There were also children under the age of nine who were supervised by the public authorities either because they were placed for reward by their parents in foster homes or were placed for adoption. Most of these categories, with the exception of the children cared for under the 1930 Poor Law Act, were in effect the result of an accumulation of protective child legislation which had begun during the second half of the nineteenth century and which had continued spasmodically up to the outbreak of the Second World War. The quality of poor law care of children had, on the whole, improved after the end of the First World War as a result of the efforts by boards of guardians to diversify methods of care. Foster homes, cottage homes, scattered homes and nurseries were used for placements, though the workhouse was still in use for a sizeable minority. Young offenders could be placed in reformatory schools (later approved schools) from the middle of the nineteenth century onwards; children found to be in need of care or protection, or young offenders, could be committed to the care of the local authority after 1933.[1] Mentally and physically handicapped children had gradually been extracted from poor law care since the commencement of national elementary education in 1870 and the beginnings of local, personal health services in the last decades of the nineteenth century. Children placed privately for reward had been protected to a limited extent from 1872 and officially supervised since 1897 and the same sort of protective supervision had been extended to some, but not all, children placed for legal adoption since 1926.[2] The newcomers to these categories were the war orphans and children left over from the massive evacuation schemes of the recent war years. In 1945 there were about 3,200 war orphans, all in foster homes and a further 850 who were being supervised in their own homes because of unsatisfactory circumstances. They were the direct responsibility of the Ministry of Pensions which employed a staff of eighteen women to concern themselves solely with the welfare of these children. The evacuees, 5,200 of them (fewer than had been forecast by the Ministry of Health), were those who were unable to return home either because they had no home to return to or because there was some other good reason for postponing their return to their parents.[3]

Altogether the Curtis Committee's review of these various categories covered a total of nearly 125,000 children and the committee quickly discovered the bewildering maze of Acts and regulations which led to the confused administration of services. Although the scene in 1945 is now of historical interest only, it is salutary to recount briefly the state into which the services had fallen.

Services for children had developed erratically, often on an *ad hoc* basis, without reference to each other. Consequently responsibility for providing or supervising substitute homes for the deprived was scattered throughout various central government departments and local authorities' committees. At central level, the Ministry of Health, the Home Office, the Board of Control, the Ministry of Education and the Ministry of Pensions were all involved and at local authority level, public assistance committees, education and health committees, the latter often acting through their maternity and child welfare committees. It all depended on the administrative category in which a child was placed, which in turn depended on such factors as why he first came to public notice, his age, whether he had been committed through the courts and so on. Perhaps the most bewildering administrative maze was that in which the poor law children found themselves. Under the Local Government Act 1929, which transferred poor law functions from local boards of guardians to county councils and county boroughs, these local authorities were required to prepare administrative schemes which provided for giving assistance where possible through social welfare legislation other than the Poor Law Acts. In the Poor Law Act, 1930, public assistance committees could delegate their functions to be discharged by any of the other committees of the council. In particular, children under the age of five, provided they were handicapped physically and mentally and ostensibly in poor law care, could be dealt with under legislation which ranged over seven Acts, the oldest being the Public Health Act 1875, and the most recent, the Education Act 1921. Other children, apart from those dealt with directly under the Poor Law Act 1930 itself, were dealt with by a mixture of central and local governments departments under a further seven enactments.

The administrative schemes in operation could hardly be described as systematic since the word 'system' implies an orderly arrangement of functions and this the organization of administration could not claim to be. The Curtis Committee,[4] in their efforts to disentangle the skein, had plenty of comments to make about the administration of child care functions of which only a few examples can be noted here: the Ministry of Health was responsible for supervising the work of local authorities in providing for those destitute children covered by the poor law. Such children could however also be accepted into homes run by voluntary organizations independently of any public authority, in which case, if the voluntary organization concerned received subscriptions from the public, the State brought them under inspection, not through the Ministry of Health however, but through the Home Office. But it *could* bring them under the inspection of the Ministry of Health, instead of the Home Office, if the former had 'certified' the homes as suitable for poor law children or if poor law children were received in them.

Children who appeared before juvenile courts could in certain circumstances be committed to the care of the local authority in whose area they normally lived, in which case they were boarded out under rules laid down by the Home Office; but if there was difficulty in finding a foster home, they could be left in a public assistance institution, in which case the Ministry of Health became involved.

The fact that at local level the public assistance committees could delegate their functions to other committees could lead to some confusing situations. This is what the Curtis Committee found in one county borough: this town's public assistance committee retained ultimate responsibility for its cottage homes for children but the education committee was given direct responsibility for administering them. The cottage homes were closely connected with the workhouse which came under the direct supervision of the public assistance committee and shared its medical services. Commented the Curtis Committee: 'members of the two committees appeared to be in constant argument'. A child, after spending his infancy in the workhouse nursery, might be moved for a short period to the cottage homes, next to a residential nursery under the public health committee and back to the cottage homes.

Finally the education authority might be responsible for his aftercare.[5]

In December 1944 the government announced that a committee of enquiry into the care of children was to be appointed for England and Wales and in view of differences in the law, a separate committee for Scotland. The committee for England and Wales was set up jointly by the Home Secretary and the Ministers for Health and for Education in March 1945, the committee for Scotland a month later. The need for the enquiries had been prompted by a good deal of agitation by public-minded people. In July 1944, Lady Allen of Hurtwood had written to *The Times* drawing attention to the plight of homeless children and criticizing the quality of care they tended to receive by public agencies. She wrote: 'The public are, for the most part, unaware that many thousands of these children are being brought up under repressive conditions that are generations out of date and are unworthy of our traditional care for children. Many who are orphaned, destitute or neglected, still live under the chilly stigma of "charity"; too often they form groups isolated from the main stream of life and education, and few of them know the comfort and security of individual affection. In many "Homes" both charitable and public, the willing staff are, for the most part, overworked, underpaid and untrained; indeed there is no recognised system of training. Inspection ... is totally inadequate and few standards are established or expected. Because no one Government Department is fully responsible, the problem is the more difficult to tackle ...'.

Subsequent to this letter, she expanded her criticisms in a pamphlet in which she cited first-hand accounts from adults who had themselves been in care, parents who for one reason or another had been obliged to part with their children and people who had worked in various children's homes. The stories they told made sad reading. Some of the conventions adopted by certain organizations verged on the preposterous: Here are a few examples from her pamphlet:

> At one large Home that takes only illegitimate children, every child on entry is rebaptised and renamed so as to make a complete break with the parent. Mothers may 'inquire' as to their children's health and may send presents.

In another Home, she wrote,

> it is also usual practice to put children of one, two and three years in separate groups ... In such a Home for children of three years, not one of the children could talk. The matron said: 'They do not need to talk, everything is done for them'.

In yet another Home there were

> dormitories and a dining-room but no playroom and no toys or occupational apparatus, not even paper and chalks. In the dining-room there is one table with a big label 'For Pigs'.[6]

But it was her initial letter to *The Times* which sparked off a correspondence demanding a government enquiry. The country had already become acquainted with the condition of many children in the towns by virtue of the revelations of the evacuation schemes. Professor Titmuss in his study of the social services in wartime has also noted that the evacuation schemes originally designed to transfer children to safety began to take on a different role by receiving children into care from about the middle of 1941 onwards; children who were considered to be the social casualties of the times, for instance: children of mothers who were ill, expecting another baby and whose husbands were in the Services, children whose mothers were forced through shortage of income to go out to work, children from homes where there were matrimonial quarrels and suchlike situations. 'The evacuation scheme,' he says, 'designed as an integral part of civil defence, increasingly assumed the form of a social welfare agency which placed children in temporary boarding homes, or residential nurseries and hostels in various parts of the country.'[7] A study, made in the early years of the war by the Women's Group on Public Welfare, had focused on the circumstances of such children and revealed the extent and depth of the problems of the deprived child.[8] A wartime increase in illegitimate children, always a group that gets the rawest deal, had already been the subject of special attention by the Ministry of Health, which had requested local authority welfare departments to co-operate with the voluntary agencies in the supervision of such children, who tended frequently to be handed over at birth to women willing to keep them on a *de facto* adoptive basis.

There was in fact ample evidence for the need for change. In any case, the Beveridge plan concerned with social security had been presented to Parliament in November 1942 and preparations were being made for the ending of the Poor Law. The care of children would inevitably require reconsideration.

If further justification for the setting up of a committee of enquiry was needed it was amply supplied in the O'Neill case. Given a weak administrative structure of child care, sooner or later some tragedy in human terms was inevitable and in this particular case there was no doubt as to where the blame had to be laid. Briefly the circumstances were as follows: Dennis and Terence O'Neill were two of four children who had been committed to the care of Newport County Borough in 1939 on account of parental neglect. Subsequently, as was the invariable practice of this authority in these cases, they were placed with foster parents in the administrative area of Shropshire.[9] Unfortunately the foster parents ill-treated the children so much that Dennis died, as the official record put it, 'from injuries which he received in the foster home while in a state of undernourishment due to neglect'. The coroner's jury added a rider to their verdict that there had been a serious lack of supervision by the local authority. Both Newport and Shropshire asked the Home Secretary for a public enquiry into the matter. This was held under Sir Walter Monckton and a report published in May 1945. The Monckton Report showed up the muddle in administrative arrangements, failure of communication between the two authorities and lack of supervision by them of the foster home.[10]

The O'Neill case provoked strong Press reaction and the country was profoundly shocked. The grim irony of the case was that these children had originally been committed because of neglect, only to suffer this to a worse degree whilst in the care of a public authority. By the time the Monckton Report was made public the Curtis Committee was already at work.

The Curtis Report

The Curtis Committee took a bare eighteen months to complete their enquiry, from March 1945 to September 1946.[11] In this time they examined 229 witnesses, visited

451 institutions of various kinds in all parts of the country and in the course of their tours interviewed officials and members of 58 local authorities. The enquiry was the first ever in this country which had been directed specifically at the care of children deprived of a normal home life and covering all groups of such children. The chairman was Myra Curtis (later Dame Myra Curtis), principal of Newnham College, Cambridge. The scope of the Committee's work covered the public care of children, methods of care and the distribution of responsibility. What they discovered about the latter has already been discussed in this chapter. What they discovered about methods of care was hardly less disquieting than the state of distribution of responsibilities. Although the Committee pointed out that the situation was not uniformly depressing, the standards of care in many cases came in, justifiably, for harsh criticism. Residential care produced the worst examples. Children were placed in a variety of residential establishments, such as public assistance homes and nurseries, public health nurseries, voluntary organizations' homes, hostels for working boys and girls, probation hostels, approved schools, remand homes and institutions for the handicapped. A wide range of facilities offered a commensurately wide spread of quality of care. Though few homes showed abuses involving neglect or harsh usage the Committee found many examples of unsatisfactory standards, where the defects lay not so much in harshness of treatment but in dirt and dreariness, drabness and over-regimentation. In their general impression of care arrangements, the committee stated that they found many establishments under both local authority and voluntary management in which children were being brought up by unimaginative methods. In some homes, they considered the standards

to be no better, except in the matter of discipline, than those of the early years of this century—a period when, according to the minority report of the Poor Law Commission 1909, standards of child care by the Boards of Guardians were in general very low.[12] A grave fault, the Committee found, lay in the widespread shortage of the right kind of staff, qualified by temperament and training to provide the child with a good substitute for a home background. There was a lack of interest in and affection for children; the Committee commented: 'the child is not recognized as an individual with his own rights and possessions, with his own life to live but merely one of a large group submerged in it.' More important still, there was no one to whom he could turn who would meet his individual needs or who was vitally interested in his welfare. The effect of this was seen by visiting Committee members who noticed the smaller children's almost pathological clamour for attention and overt affection, and the older children's slowness, backwardness, lack of response, habits of destructiveness and lack of concentration. Where, on the other hand, individual love and care had been given, the children's behaviour was notably different, displaying no undue interest in their visitors and happily pursuing their own occupations and games.

The one type of care which the Committee found commendable was boarding-out. They had visited a number of foster homes and while they found some which for one reason or another they found unsuitable, there were few in which the child was not accepted as a member of the household or failed to find affection and happiness. In their conclusions on boarding-out, they considered that although there was probably a risk of unhappiness in a foster home, and of course they were well aware of the O'Neill case, a happy foster home was far preferable to life as generally lived in a large residential community,[13] and 'large' was the right adjective to apply to some of the public assistance homes which were of the 'barrack' type, built during the nineteenth century and housing two hundred children or more.

It was evident to the Committee that what was urgently required was a re-allocation of administrative responsibility for deprived children in a much more simplified and unitary structure. Many of the care problems, breakdowns of communication, failures to allocate responsibility and kindred problems stemmed from this lack.

Another area of concern was the absence in many cases of the quality of personal attention which deprived children require; the Committee were concerned to make the care service a much more personal one for the children.

A third area which needed consideration was whether public responsibility covered a wide enough field: whether there were groups of children needing care or supervision who were beyond its scope.

All three problems were covered in the recommendations. The main recommendations can be summarized under three headings:

1. Central responsibility for all deprived children should be vested in one government department and an advisory council on child care should be appointed.
2. Local responsibility should be exercised by a new children's committee at county council and county borough level to take over the care functions previously exercised by other committees.
3. The new committee should be served by a children's officer with chief officer status, who would have his

own department dealing solely with the care of deprived children.

On the subject of central responsibility, the Curtis Committee had to consider whether a single department should be responsible for every aspect of the life of a deprived child, e.g. education, health and so on. To do so would have emphasized his 'separateness' from other children and this they particularly wished to minimize. After all, they argued, these children were different only in respect of one missing element in their lives and that was in the normality of their home life. What they needed was someone to take on the parental role.

The Committee decided against nominating one of the eligible central departments for this role. 'Which department', they said, 'is a question which must be settled on another level, and it does not seem to us to be so important as the achievement of unification.'[14]

As for local responsibility, the Committee was only too well aware of the confusion of functions. The situation called for reform. No one felt actively and personally responsible for the welfare of individual children, and arguments between committees as to who should foot the bill for care left the child in the meantime without proper care. There had been a good deal of evidence supplied by the local authorities themselves that this division of functions was harmful to good child care practice and that one committee only should undertake the work. But which one? There the witnesses parted company, except that it was generally accepted that it should not be the public assistance committee. It seems likely from the evidence of the interest groups concerned that they supported their own stake in the status quo, were resistant to any suggestion of radical change, and did not see the need for it. The prospect of administrative reform called into question their competence and threatened their future. In fact, except for the evidence submitted by the central departments, the one common characteristic of the evidence from the interest groups was that it stated the case of the organization presenting it.[15] Arguments advanced by the education groups, for example, were to the effect that the whole work relating to children over the age of two should be handed to the local education committees since the Education Act 1944 already entrusted them with the education of all children over that age and empowered them to provide residential accommodation. For infants under two, the maternity and child welfare committees could take responsibility since they already provided residential nurseries. The Curtis Committee had two serious objections to these proposals: one was that this sort of scheme would still require a transfer of responsibility for a child at a time in his life when it was vitally important that he should have continuity of care, of surroundings and of human relations; secondly the child care functions, if left in the hands of one of the existing departments, would not constitute their *primary* function; education committees, for example, were *primarily* concerned with education of the mind rather than the care of children.

The recommendation therefore was for the establishment of an *ad hoc* committee reporting direct to the council of the local authority. This committee, to be called the children's committee, would assume the responsibilities that had up to then fallen to the local authority in respect of children not in their own homes under the Poor Law Act, the Public Health Act, the Children and Young Persons Act, and the Adoption of Children Act. It would become

responsible for the boarding out of children and for provision of residential accommodation in children's homes,
approved schools and remand homes.

The proposal for the appointment of a children's officer
was linked with that for the establishment of a children's
committee. It arose from the need that the new department serving that committee should have its own executive
officer with the standing of a senior administrative official
of the council, in direct touch with his committee and not
subservient to any other chief officer. So important did
the Curtis Committee consider this appointment to be that
they suggested that in those local authorities where the
numbers of children to be dealt with were too small to
warrant a separate appointment, children's boards of
neighbouring authorities should join together under a
single children's officer to exercise all the required functions.

The Committee spelt out the kind of children's officer
they envisaged: a person of high academic qualifications,
if possible a graduate who also possessed a social science
diploma; preferably over thirty on initial appointment,
genial and friendly in manner, able to set both children
and adults at ease, with a strong interest in the welfare of
children and with enough faith and enthusiasm to be ready
to experiment with methods old and new of compensating
by care and affection those who had a bad start in life. In
conceptual terms this meant that the children's officer
would stand as a symbol for the personal element in the
relationship between the local authority and the deprived
child.

These recommendations constituted only a small part
of the report. They have been selected because they have
had far-reaching effects on the subsequent development

of child care services. There were other important recommendations, sixty-two altogether, covering such matters as the registration and inspection of voluntary organizations dealing with children, the establishment of a central department child care inspectorate, the establishment of training courses for child care staff (or boarding-out visitors, as they were then called) and the extension of categories of children who would in future need to come under public supervision, such as privately fostered children over the age of nine.

The recommendations of the Curtis Committee were accepted by the government, the Prime Minister making a statement to this effect in Parliament on 24 March, 1947. The Children Bill was introduced in the House of Lords in December of that year, but even before that time the government was able to take action on those recommendations which did not have to await special legislation, and on 24 July the Transfer of Functions (Relief of Children) Order 1947 was made under the Ministers of the Crown (Transfer of Functions) Act 1946. This enabled the responsibilities of the Minister of Health exercisable under the Poor Law Act 1930, with respect to children deprived of a normal home life, to be transferred to the Home Office. The choice of the Home Office as the Ministry with central responsibility had also been announced by the Prime Minister at the time of signifying acceptance of the Curtis recommendations. The reasons for this choice have never been made public but may be surmised. There already existed a tradition of child care functions in this Ministry. Through its historic responsibility for the administration of prisons, it had gained central control of reformatory and industrial schools as far back as the middle of the nineteenth century, and since then had gradually expanded its control and interests in all matters relating to juvenile delinquency and endangered children. It therefore had a claim to the allocation of responsibility for deprived children.[16]

The debates in Parliament on the Children Bill were of a non-political nature. This was not entirely fortuitous; the Curtis Committee had been set up by the coalition government and if blame attached for governmental negligence of duty towards deprived children then all political parties had a share in it. A major area of discussion arose from the proposal that Parliament should have the power to impose a uniform system of administration throughout the country. What was involved here was the degree of freedom local authorities could have in devising their own child care services according to the dictates of local needs, knowledge and traditions. There was a marked reluctance to submit to central control. Freedom from central control had always been of importance to local authorities, and since it would be they, rather than central government, who would have to organize and run the local services, their claim to autonomy had point; but the arguments which the Curtis Committee had put forward on this issue, namely the real need for uniformity of administrative structure, were strong, and the government was not inclined to give way. As to the establishment of a new and separate committee at local authority level, strong opposition came from the education lobby in Parliament, again, as had been argued before the Curtis Committee, on the grounds that the welfare tradition in education made the local education committee the natural executants of the Curtis ideas. Again the arguments were refuted on the grounds that, however wide education might cast its net, it always left room for the parental role and this was to be the very role that the new committee would be required to play.[17]

The Home Office lost no time in setting about the task of reorganization before the Children Bill became law. On 1 September, 1947, it invited local authorities to proceed with the formation of children's committees and the appointment of children's officers in advance of legislation. In July of that year, the Central Training Council in Child Care was appointed by the Home Secretary and in co-operation with the universities, local education authorities and voluntary organizations, training courses for child care workers were inaugurated.

The Children Bill passed its final stages at the end of June 1948 and the Act came into operation on 5 July, 1948. On that same day the National Assistance Act became law, bringing an end to the Poor Law, which had dominated social welfare provisions for the past 350 years.

The poor law care of children had a notoriously chequered history. It had its periods of harshness, even callousness, but it also had its time of humanitarianism and enlightened approach to the care of deprived children, largely due to the efforts of devoted individuals like Hannah Archer and Elisabeth Twining. But the essence of poor law policy was still expressed as late as 1946 in the Poor Law Act 1930: local authorities were charged 'to set to work or put out as apprentices all children whose parents are not, in the opinion of the Council, able to keep and maintain their children'. The Curtis Committee had pointed out that no general duties regarding education and welfare were laid upon local authorities by the Poor Law Act.

Provisions of the Children Act 1948

In order to emphasize the break with poor law traditions, it was necessary to express the new ideology of care in the Act of 1948. This was done in Section 12 and since it was to be the guiding spirit which should imbue the new children's committees it is worth quoting in full:

> Where a child is in the care of a local authority, it shall be the duty of that authority to exercise their powers with respect to him so as to further his best interests and to afford him opportunity for the proper development of his character and abilities.
>
> In providing for a child in their care, a local authority shall make use of facilities and services available to children in the care of their parents as appears to the local authority reasonable in his case.

The first part of this section emphasizes the parental role of the local authority and the second part enjoins avoidance of any kind of segregation from other children in the community.

Section 1 of the Act is concerned with the duty of the local authority of receiving into care any child under the age of seventeen in their area who for a wide variety of reasons may require it, provided the local authority considers intervention on his behalf to be in the interests of his welfare. It also makes it clear that his period in care should last only so long as his welfare requires and the local authority must endeavour to discharge him from care, if and when they consider this to be consistent with his welfare. In any case they cannot refuse to discharge him from care to his parents or legal guardians if they demand this unless the local authority have themselves obtained parental rights amounting to custody, either through a court order or a special assumption of parental rights provision under the Children Act. But for these exceptions, the imperative to return the child to his parents stems from the fact that the Children Act does not empower the local authority to receive a child into care *against the wishes* of his parents and therefore, in common justice, they should not have the power to refuse to return him to them if they demand it, so long as the parents have retained parental rights. Reception into care rests essentially upon voluntary agreement between the parents and the local authority.[18]

Local authorities were also given the *duty* to act as fit person to any child committed to their care by a court. Hitherto they had a right to refuse, and committals to local authority care remained under-used until after 1948.[19]

The care provisions which local authorities have to make were made quite explicit. Following closely on the Curtis recommendations, boarding-out, or foster care, to give its modern name, was given first priority and only if it was not desirable or practicable *for the time being* to make arrangements for fostering, could children be placed in residential establishments such as children's homes or voluntary homes. Another particular duty laid on the local authority was that of providing separate accommodation for the temporary reception of children, with facilities for the observation of their physical and mental condition. The need for adequate reception facilities was another point which had been stressed in the Curtis report as a result of the lessons learnt from the evacuation experience, although the nature of the need was going to change. At one time reception was used to ensure that the child was free from infection, now the emphasis would be placed more on diagnosis of his psychological needs.

Another section underlined the continuing responsibility of parents for children in care, since they were obliged to contribute towards their support and also had to keep in touch with the local authority. This was of course not a new provision. It amounted to a continuation of existing policy.

The appointment of an *ad hoc* children's committee and the appointment of a children's officer, the latter subject to Home Office approval, were made mandatory and the functions which the committee had to discharge were specified as arising out of particular enactments apart from which the committee were not to undertake any other work. This emphasized the principle that child care was to be not just the *primary* but the *only* function of the children's committee.

Central control was written in with the sections that local authorities were to carry out their functions under the general guidance of the Home Secretary, and the provision of an Advisory Council on Child Care.[20]

The Children Act 1948 represented a new deal for deprived children. It was then, and remains today, an important piece of social legislation. It expresses social policy towards a group of children who have lost, or are in danger of losing, the prop of a normal home life. Its advent in 1948 was inevitable. In spirit it was matched by the other great pieces of social legislation of that period, in education, health, social security and urban renewal, all of which took as their starting point the desire to create a better life for the community as a whole after the bitterness of economic depression in the twenties and thirties and the nightmare of the Second World War.

It had to come too because of the public disquiet

aroused through the revelations of evacuating hundreds of thousands of children in the forties and also because the Poor Law was doomed and damned for what it had done to thousands of families, particularly in the inter-war years, whose one fault had been the inability to find work. Ironically a new child care service might have come forty years sooner if the recommendations of the minority report of the Poor Law Commission 1909 had been taken up;[21] but in the end it was recognized that an entirely new service, created in its own right, was necessary; after all, even the minority report of 1909 had visualized its being tacked on to an existing service, i.e. education. It must also be counted as a tribute that the Children Act has undergone no major modification in the course of more than two decades.

The provisions of the Act brought together a number of functions scattered over a wide administrative field. Nevertheless even today welfare functions for children are far from unified.

Child care in the social services

In 1948, the newly organized service was charged with responsibility for the needs of the child deprived of a normal home life. The phrase, 'deprived of a normal home life' came from the terms of reference to the Curtis Committee. The Committee was specifically directed to 'inquire into existing methods of providing for children who from loss of parents or from any other cause whatever are deprived of a normal home life with their own parents or relatives'.

It was relatively easy for the Committee to define the term 'child' in the remit, since they could take account of the various legal definitions which were to be found scattered amongst a number of statutes,[22] but it was, and still remains, less easy to define in unequivocal terms what is meant by the phrase 'deprived of a normal home life', for the difficulty of applying any objective test to establish the normality of home life is immediately evident. In practice, a normal home life is discernible only on the basis of subjective judgments. The Curtis Committee did not attempt an abstraction of the term. Instead they fell back on grouping together various categories of children in whose cases the State had intervened in the interest of their welfare and for whom it had, with a few exceptions, assumed temporary or permanent care and responsibility. They also included children who were in the care of voluntary organizations or placed by parents in the care of private persons either on a fostering basis or with a view to legal adoption. The committee were not asked to enquire, nor did they enquire, into the situation of those children who could be considered 'deprived of a normal home life' while yet remaining with their parents. They were only too well aware of the existence of children in such circumstances and they raised the important question, as others had done before them, whether deprivation arising out of neglect at home, malnutrition, or other social problems might not in fact be preventable. But since this issue lay outside their terms of reference they considered that they should not at that time deal with it. Since that time the issue has been taken up and resources have been concentrated on preventive work; this matter will be discussed later in this book.

The Curtis Committee's view of deprivation was perforce a narrow one confined to the categories of children into whose circumstances they enquired. In 1948, the child care service was intended in the main as a care service for children removed from home because of deprivation. Over the years the service has gradually been extended to deal with children whose circumstances are such that a breakdown of care at home is likely to occur. In particular, since 1963, it has been able to help families with young children who are experiencing difficulties such as marital disharmony, physical or mental illness and inability to manage because of poor housing or low income; all factors which may have an adverse effect on children. The service is thus much more broadly based now than it was formerly. Although its objectives still include the care of children deprived of a normal home life, it has become much more an all-purpose child welfare service; but it does not have a monopoly in the field of child welfare, even its specific care functions are shared to some extent with other social services.

Two of these, at the local authority level, are the education and health services. Both, in point of fact, carried some functions which they gave up to the newly formed child care service, but they retained others.

The education service has a long tradition in the welfare field. G. A. N. Lowndes, the education historian, has commented that nationals of other countries often find some difficulty in understanding why the public service of education accepts responsibility for so many welfare ser‧ vices.[23] The reasons may be found partly in the fact that soon after elementary education was made compulsory on a national scale, in 1876, teachers and other educationalists considered it pointless to force even a rudimentary education on children, many of whom were too undernourished, ill-clad or fatigued to derive any advantage from it. The teachers' concern led in time to the introduction of school meals and the medical inspection of all children on commencing their schooling.

Today the welfare functions of school meals and medical inspection remain, together with the provision of clothing in necessitous cases to enable children to attend school. Apart from this, the education service has a responsibility for providing special education for a variety of handicapped children in special day or boarding schools or in special units attached to normal schools. The welfare aspect of education is well epitomized in these provisions. About two-thirds of maladjusted children have to be educated in special boarding schools. The child care service often provides care facilities for these children and there is a good deal of overlap of provision between the two services. Since the publication of the report of the Plowden committee on primary education,[24] the linking of school and home has been given fresh attention. The committee commissioned research and used published material which showed the extent to which home and neighbourhood conditions affect children's educational progress. It emphasized the need for the creation or expansion of many kinds of school welfare functions.[25]

The health service has a similar record of seventy or so years' effort in the field of child welfare. The local authority personal health services, apart from providing treatment facilities for school-age children referred to them by the school health service, were largely concerned in the first decades of this century with the care of mothers and their young children. The reason for their concern with this particular group lay in the disquiet caused by the persistence of a high incidence of infant mortality,[26] compared with a general death rate which was declining. Over the years the service has greatly expanded its scope of operations by providing services for adults, but a strong emphasis on the medical and social care of infants remains through the provision of clinics for maternity and infant welfare day nurseries, supervision of child minding and health visiting to advise mothers on the care of their pre-school age children. In some areas local health authorities undertake work with problem families and give help to unmarried mothers and their children.

Through their mental health functions, health departments also provide such specialized services for children as training centres for sub-normal or severely sub-normal children (although training centres for children are in process of being transferred to education departments, as a result of a recommendation by the Seebohm committee).

The sources of child welfare functions are liberally spread around the statutory services. Apart from the local authority services mentioned so far, they include the probation service and the police.

The probation service was created in its modern statutory form in the early years of this century and since then has worked extensively in the child welfare field. Although its activities are best known for the supervision of persons referred on court orders, it has fulfilled other functions in recent years. Probation officers have worked in welfare enquiries, the supervision of children involved in the matrimonial disputes and matrimonial proceedings of their parents, the supervision of children who come before juvenile courts because of cruelty and neglect, and in adoption procedures. In the future its new status as the 'Probation and After-Care Service' implies a shift to concentration on work with adults, but for the time being it has a prominent part to play in the child welfare field.

The contribution of the police in the context of this

discussion is not generally known, the police are not normally classified as a social service; yet for a number of years, some police forces have been running juvenile liaison schemes. These involve children and young persons who might otherwise have to be brought before a juvenile court. Specially selected police officers carry out welfare-cum-preventive functions to ensure that youngsters do not get into trouble with the law. Although the number of children involved in any one area is usually small, success in places like Liverpool, which inaugurated police-juvenile liaison about twenty years ago, has gradually led to the adoption of similar schemes in a number of forces including the Metropolitan Police.

Apart from the statutory services, voluntary organizations continue to play their part as they have done for more than a century. Today, less numerous than they were, they still form an integral part of the welfare front.[27] The statutory services rely on them to supplement their own work, experiment with new methods for dealing with problems and to fill the gaps which inevitably appear through the uneven distribution of statutory resources. In many instances, a voluntary organization is financed or partly financed by a local authority to carry out a particular statutory function, but in other cases it will rely on its own resources for its work. Some of the better-known ones have made reputations for themselves in specialist fields of child welfare. Amongst them are organizations like the N.S.P.C.C. which has been campaigning on behalf of cruelly treated and neglected children for ninety years and the Invalid Children's Aid Society which has for decades given assistance to handicapped children and their families.

The extension of child welfare services has intensified

the demands made on voluntary organizations. In successive Acts of Parliament concerned with child welfare their contribution has been recognized and, whatever the pattern of future services, they are unlikely to be dispensed with.[28]

The reason why these services are cited is that many of the functions carried out by the specifically designated child care service are also being carried out by other statutory and voluntary services. For example: at the present time the child care service makes arrangements for the care of maladjusted children—so does the education service; it carries out a preventive service to safeguard illegitimate children—so does the health service; it supervises children who are brought to public notice because of parental neglect—so does the probation service; it is engaged in child-delinquency prevention—so are the police; it provides a care service for children away from their families and makes arrangements for adoptions—so do the various voluntary organizations.

The Committee on Local Authority and Allied Personal Social Services (1968) recommended a rationalization of the child welfare functions of various agencies and we shall take up this point again later; for the purpose of this chapter it must be reiterated that child welfare functions are often interwoven with the other functions carried out by major social service agencies.

Notes

1. The first legislation which enabled a court to entrust the care care of young offenders to suitable persons was passed in 1840, the Infant Felons Act. Its object was 'to remove children from the influence of vicious parents'. It proved to be an ineffectual measure.

2. The development of child care has been documented by J. S. Heywood, *Children in Care*, Routledge & Kegan Paul, second edition, 1965.

3. R. M. Titmuss, *Problems of Social Policy*, H.M.S.O. and Longmans, p. 437. The Ministry of Health had forecast that about 10,000 evacuated children would be left without a home to which to return.

4. *Report of the Care of Children Committee* (Curtis), 1946, Cmnd. 6922.

5. *Ibid.*, para. 120.

6. Marjory, Baroness Allen of Hurtwood, *Whose Children?* On the condition of children brought up in charitable homes, institutions, etc., p. 32. Distributed Simpkin Marshall, London 1945.

7. Titmuss, *op. cit.*, pp. 404-5.

8. Women's Group on Public Welfare, *Our Towns—A Close up*, O.U.P., 1943.

9. This apparently was common practice. Liverpool, for instance, in 1939, had entered into close reciprocal arrangements with the education departments of other authorities, e.g. Derbyshire, Leicester, Bolton, etc., for the exchange of foster homes. Liverpool's children were almost invariably boarded out in the area of another local authority, large families being split up between two or more neighbouring foster homes. See *Then and Now 1949-1963*, Report on the Work, Organization and Development of the Liverpool Children's Department, p. 18.

10. *Report on the Boarding out of Dennis and Terence O'Neill 1945-46*, Cmnd. 6636 (Monckton Report).

11. The Curtis committee issued an Interim Report in March 1946, Cmnd. 6760, on the subject of training in child care.

12. J. Parker, *Local Authority Health and Welfare Services*, Allen & Unwin, 1965, pp. 22-23.

13. Curtis Report, paras. 415-422.

14. *Ibid.*, para. 434.

15. J. Warham, 'The History of the Children Bill in a County Borough 1946-48'. Unpublished M.A. thesis, University of Liverpool, 1965, Ch. II.

16. The Ministry of Health and the Ministry of Education, it could be argued, had equally strong claims. They may not have pressed these too far in view of the fact that each was fully extended with implementing recently passed legislation, the Education Act, 1944 and the National Health Services Act, 1946, respectively.

17. For a fuller discussion of these issues, see J. Warham, *op. cit.*

18. There are times when the local authority, the police or the N.S.P.C.C. may have to remove a child from a neglectful home against the wishes of the parents. In such cases action would have to be taken under a statute such as the Children and Young Persons Act 1933-69.

19. See P. Boss, 'Children Committed to Care—The Development and Use of the Fit Person Order', *Child Care*, Vol. XX, No. 3, October 1966.

20. A fuller discussion of the main provisions of the Children Act 1948 can be found in Heywood, *op. cit.*, ch. 9.

21. J. Parker, *op. cit.*, ch. 11.

22. The Committee found that different Acts of Parliament defined a child variously as a person up to 14, 18 and 21 years old. They decided not to regard themselves bound by any particular age limit.

23. G. A. N. Lowndes, *The English Educational System*, Hutchinson, 1960, p. 119.

24. *Children and Their Primary Schools*, H.M.S.O., 1966.

25. The need for school welfare services is argued in: A. Clegg and B. Megson, *Children in Distress*, Penguin, 1968.

26. Infant mortality rate (i.e. death rate of infants under one year of age per thousand children born) in 1900 was 154, in 1914 it was 105. In 1918 came the first Maternity and Child Welfare Act and by 1928 the rate had dropped to 69. At present it is 18.3.

27. *Report on the Work of the Children's Department, Home Office 1964-66*, pp. 13-15.

28. On this point see D. Owen, *English Philanthropy*, O.U.P., 1964, p. 533.

3

The Children Act in operation

Starting the service

Even before the Children Act 1948 came into operation, the Home Secretary was able to tell Parliament in June of that year that in anticipation of the Act sixty local authorities had already appointed separate children's committees.[1] This was interpreted as an indication of the readiness of local authorities to accept the administrative framework about to be thrust on them by legislation, but whether it was keenness to get started on the new enterprise or resignation in the face of the inevitable is a moot point. The Home Office claimed that the transfer of functions to the newly established children's departments from existing ones was carried through smoothly and that by the end of 1948 the new arrangements were taking satisfactory shape.[2] An indication of the willingness of a few local authorities to get started can be gauged from their departmental reports: Lancashire County Council is on record as saying that their children's committee was appointed in 1946 (actually six months before the Curtis Committee itself was set up).[3] Cheshire County Council claims to have been 'first in the field' with a fully fledged children's welfare and care department and designated children's welfare officer commencing their work on

1 April 1947.[4] Others took longer. In Liverpool the newly-formed children's committee held its first meeting on 1 September 1948 but the appointment of the children's officer did not become effective for a further six months and it was not until eight months after the appointed day that the city children's department came into existence.[5] Birmingham's children's department, complete with children's officer, began operations on 1 February 1949 but a considerable length of time elapsed before all the functions due to the new department could be transferred from their former department and it was July 1950 before this change-over was completed.[6]

Altogether there were 143 local authorities with children's committees. A few authorities had taken advantage of the provision in the Children Act which enabled two or more local authorities to appoint the same person to be children's officer for each of them. In one instance three authorities appointed the same person. In these cases a small authority joined forces with a larger neighbour, as for example, Canterbury and Kent. These various local authority areas which had now become children's authorities served contrastingly sized populations. The largest was the London County Council with a population, in 1949, of around 3,389,000, and other similarly huge local authorities were Lancashire and Middlesex with populations exceeding two million and West Riding of Yorkshire, Essex, Kent and Surrey and Birmingham with over one million each. At the other end of the population scale were Radnorshire with little more than 20,000, Merionethshire (41,000) and Montgomeryshire (48,000). The point was that with the exception of the local authorities which decided to form a joint service with a larger neighbour, each county and county borough, however small, had full autonomy over its service, and from the outset it could be said to be that many of them were too small for the efficient running of a child care service.[7]

Numbers in care

The varying numbers of children in care of local authorities reflected the varying sizes of population in their areas. At the end of 1952, for example, the total number in care of all authorities in England and Wales was 64,682. The share of the large local authorities already mentioned was respectively: 8,027, 1,599, 2,727, 1,890, 1,487, 2,187, 1,464 and 1,503, and of the small authorities: 40, 43 and 39 respectively.

There were also substantial differences between local authorities in the number of children in care expressed as a proportion of the child population under eighteen in each area. The average for all areas in 1952, for example, was 5·6 per 1,000; but this average included the figures for Cardiganshire (12·1); Bournemouth (10·8); London (10·4); and Reading (10·1) at one extreme and Northumberland, Wallasey, Montgomeryshire, each with 3·2 at the other extreme. Why there should be these variations, which have persisted to the present, has not yet been satisfactorily explained.[8]

The number of children in care rose substantially during the first few years of the life of the new service—by 18% between 1949 and 1953. In 1946 the Curtis Committee had estimated that local authorities had about 46,000 children in their care—exact statistics were not available. Demographic changes no doubt had some bearing on the increased numbers in care; the rise in the birth rate just after the war had the effect of adding more children to

Table 1

Number of Children in Care and Received and Discharged 1949-1959, England and Wales

Year ending	Total number in care	Rate p. 1,000 of estimated population under 18	Number of children received into care	Number of children discharged from care
30 November 1949	55,255	—	—	—
1950	58,987	—	33,927	29,674
1951	62,691	—	36,590	32,786
1952	64,682	5·6	37,977	36,002
1953	65,309	5·4	39,300	38,647
1954	64,560	5·5	39,498	40,247
31 March 1956	62,347	5·3	38,120	39,422
1957	62,033	5·2	39,096	39,410
1958	62,070	5·2	40,021	39,979
1959	61,580	5·1	40,319	40,806

the population potentially at risk. But what the Children Act had done was to open the door to care much wider than before. It also brought with it a new spirit of service. Children's committees were able to interpret the Act in a liberal way and soon uncovered social needs, previously hidden, which their departments could now meet. The number of children received into care rose steadily until 1965.

Discharges from care every year also rose commensurate with receptions. This suggested a rapid turnover of a sizeable proportion of children in care. Confirmation of this came in a study made for the Home Office by the Social Survey Division of the Central Office of Information for 1956 and 1957.[9] It showed, amongst other things, that the proportion of children coming into care on a given day who would still be in care after a period of six weeks was about 50%, after one year 23%, after two years 19% and after five years 11%. Put another way it meant that about two-thirds of the children who came into care during a year would leave care again before its ending and that the one-third who remained represented about one-fifth of the total number in care at the end of the year, the remaining four-fifths being made up of children who had already been in care for one or more years. The turnover of large numbers of 'short-term' children reduced the average stay in care to 1¾ years, but the majority of children in care at any one time were, and still are, those who have been in care for four or more years. Major reasons for the short-term intake proved to be due to temporary illness or confinement of the mother. Children's departments quickly found themselves involved in this short-term work which had not been fully anticipated either by the Curtis Committee or the Home Office.

One aspect of child care which had been heavily under lined in the Children Act was the need for the early rehabilitation of children in care with their parents. Substitute care with the local authority was seen as only second best to the child living with his own family. There was of course no problem with short-term children; but with the long-term children very often the reasons that brought them into care meant that an early return home, or even return at all, was in doubt. Children were coming into long-term care because they had been orphaned, because they had been deserted or the home had broken up for other reasons, because a parent, more often the mother, was suffering from a chronic mental disorder, or had been imprisoned. A grave shortage of housing, particularly in the early years of the child care service, also hampered efforts of rehabilitation, and a steady stream of children committed to care by juvenile courts meant in many cases that home conditions were too adverse to allow them to remain.[10] Child care staff were too few in numbers to cope with the extensive efforts involved in improving home conditions to enable children to return. Rehabilitation sometimes happened spontaneously; in other cases, it was difficult or impossible to achieve.

The sixties saw a sizeable expansion in the work of children's departments. The implementation of the preventive-work functions of the Children and Young Persons Act 1963, which will be discussed in greater detail later in this book, imposed a considerable additional amount of work, but there were other functions, less publicized, which reached more and more people: adoption work, child protection duties and approved school after-care functions. There was also the rise in the number of children who came into care via fit person orders, which indicates that children's departments were being drawn more and more into contact with the juvenile courts, and to a lesser extent with other courts since the advent of the Matrimonial Proceedings Acts of 1958 and 1960. Hopes that the preventive functions would result in the reduction of the number of children in care did not materialize until 1968, when for the first time in the decade the numbers in care were marginally less than in the previous year. In 1967 they had reached the highest point since such statistics were first recorded in 1949. More significantly, the 1968 figures showed a quite substantial reduction in the number of children *received* into care during the course of the year.

Table 2 illustrates the trends from 1960 to 1968.

The number of children in care on one day in 1968 was about 13% higher than the number for the same day in 1960, and there was a slight percentage increase in the rate of children in care expressed as a proportion of the population under 18. It should be borne in mind that the number of children in the care of voluntary organizations has dropped over the years since 1960, and this exacerbated a situation in which the local authorities were faced with increasing numbers year by year. The rise in the number of children received into care each year reached its peak in 1965 when it stood 30% above the 1960 figure.

The factors which govern care statistics, as we have already noted, are highly complex. Ronald Walton, who has made a special study of these statistics, correlates rising numbers since 1960 with an increase in the population considered to be at risk, suggesting that this reflects higher expectations by society of the quality of child rearing standards in families.[11] There is some evidence for this in an analysis made by the Home Office on changes in the primary reasons for children coming into care over a

Table 2

Number of Children in Care and Received and Discharged 1960 to 1968, England and Wales

Year ending 31 March	Total number of children in care	Rate p. 1,000 of estimated population under 18	Number of children received into care	Number of children discharged from care
1960	61,729	5·0	42,048	41,900
1961	62,199	5·0	45,203	44,754
1962	63,648	5·1	47,471	46,019
1963	64,807	5·1	48,479	47,319
1964	66,281	5·1	51,810	50,337
1965	67,099	5·1	54,659	53,637
1966	69,157	5·3	54,471	52,457
1967	69,405	5·3	53,381	53,187
1968	69,358	5·2	50,938	50,919

three year period. It was noted that rises in 1965-6 compared with 1962-3 were particularly marked in cases of children abandoned or lost—up by 50%, desertions by mother—up by 31%, unsatisfactory home conditions—up by 81%, the only circumstance in which there was a decrease, by a third, was in cases of children made homeless through eviction.[12]

The effect of the increase in work on children's departments can be gauged from a recently published Home Office Research Unit report.[13] This revealed that half of the working time of a child care officer was spent on children in care and just under a quarter was taken up with preventive work and dealing with applications to care, the remaining quarter being widely spread over other types of work.

Before a child could be received into care his family circumstances had to be investigated. In the early fifties, the number of children referred for care was usually about twice the number eventually received into care. Enquiries were often extensive and protracted. The Eighth Report of the Home Office Children's Department, commenting on this, spoke of the long and intensive casework which was often necessary to enable a family to keep together and maintain a reasonable mode of living. It was not just a question of the cost of the care involved. Time spent on a family in difficulty, primarily in the interests of children, could mean in the long run that the children did not repeat their parents' mistakes; and in the short term it helped to reduce the demand which the parents made on the services of the community.[14] Child care officers soon ran into the thick of family problems and many times it must have seemed easier to cut through the Gordian knot of the difficulties and receive the children into care, to extract at least some of them from thoroughly unsatisfactory situations, than to embark on the arduous task of keeping the family together. Prior to 1963 it was doubtful how far staff time and other resources could legally be devoted to this sort of preventive action. The Children Act itself was silent on this point, but a Home Office circular on the Act which had been issued to children's authorities in 1948 stressed the importance of doing all that was possible to save children from becoming deprived, and suggested that where a home could be improved to make it unnecessary to remove a child, or where a child who had been removed could be restored to his parents' care, this course of action should be pursued.[15] But local authorities had to be mindful of the questions the district auditor would ask if he found expenditure on work for which statutory authority could not be cited.

The preventive approach was more than a common-sense exercise. Dr Bowlby's classic monograph,[16] based on mother-child separation theory, quoted a considerable body of empirical evidence indicating the adverse effects which could follow when infants were separated from their mothers. Infants and young children, the message went, need to experience a warm, intimate and continuous relationship with their mothers or permanent mother substitutes in order to safeguard their future mental health. The implication was that child care officers, receiving children into care with the best of motives, might actually be instrumental in endangering the children's future mental health. The monograph, published for the World Health Organization, came out in 1951, and although later studies somewhat modified the theory, for the time being it gave full encouragement to the child care service to prevent separation. Despite the best efforts of residential workers and foster parents, it was difficult to ensure an adequate, permanent mother substitute for young children coming into care. The Social Survey study, referred to earlier in this chapter, showed too that nearly one-fifth of children coming into care were under one year old at the time, though evidently many stayed in care for a relatively brief period only, and Dr Bowlby's study was directed more at the dangers resulting from long-term separation.

The cost of care was a further powerful factor encouraging preventive work. In 1954, the Association of Children's Officers' Bulletin reprinted an article from *The Economist* in which some comparative cost figures were cited. 'The weekly cost of infants in public nurseries', it said, 'is frequently between 10 and 11 guineas which is higher than fees at Eton ... one family of four children who were in care over six years cost a local authority close on £7,000'. It then continued to give some examples of successful work done by London County Council relating to family support preventing receptions into care—'experiments ... undertaken despite the Children Act, rather than because of it.'[17]

But nearly ten more years were to elapse before the necessary legal sanction for preventive work was granted.

Problems of accommodation

The pressure on the young service exerted by the annually rising turnover of cases and expanding numbers of children in care was increased by the resultant pressure on accommodation. Much of the residential accommodation which children's departments up and down the country had inherited was badly outdated. It fell into five general categories:

1. Family Group Homes:
   These accommodated usually not more than twelve children in an ordinary house in an ordinary residential street, the idea being to simulate as closely as possible a normal, if rather large, family house. Normally such homes were staffed by a residential housemother and an assistant.

2. Grouped Cottage Homes:
   These consisted of a group of cottages, usually adjacent to each other, each housing from 10 to 20 children in the charge of a housemother plus an assistant or else a married couple.

3. Large Homes:
   Larger than family group homes and not organized as cottage homes, varying in size, the biggest (around 1950) accommodated as many as 480 children. There was a commensurately large staff headed by a superintendent and matron, a married couple holding a joint appointment.

4. Residential Nurseries:
   There was a large stock of nurseries left over from Poor Law days, many of them placed close to the public assistance institution and commonly in use for the under-fives. The number of children they accommodated varied, the largest, according to the Sixth Report of the Home Office Children's Department, housing 185 children.

5. Reception Centres:
   There were only a few of these, since for reception purposes, prior to the Children Act, local authorities housed children temporarily in public assistance institutions for cleansing and treatment of skin diseases and

other minor ailments, before placing them in children's homes.

In addition a few local authorities had hostels for working boys. The Children Act was explicit about the kinds of establishment which would be used for residential accommodation. In particular it stressed the need for separate reception facilities with facilities for observation of children's physical and mental condition. The Home Office issued a special memorandum of guidance to local authorities on the subject of providing reception facilities for children likely to stay in care for more than six months, and in the first three periodic reports on local authorities child care work, featured reception facilities and reception centres quite extensively. In point of fact local authorities responded well to the duty of provision. There were almost no facilities in 1948, but 60 reception centres were in operation by the end of 1954 and 85 in 1960. Of these 30 provided full facilities for making assessment, calling on the services of a psychologist or psychiatrist as necessary.

The uphill task which faced children's departments in tackling their residential accommodation shortages can be gauged from the Home Office Report of 1951. On cottage Homes: 'In many ... the number of staff are inadequate, with the result that housemothers are harassed and overworked and are unable to give the children the personal interest they need ... the standard of furnishing in cottage homes is gradually improving, but there is still in some a general drabness which, combined with the depressing buildings, gives them an institutional appearance'. On large Homes: 'The biggest of the buildings are institutional in character and are an embarrassing legacy to authorities anxious to develop the care of children on modern lines. The characteristics of these Homes are large dormitories and playrooms which in themselves constitute an insuperable obstacle to the creation of a homelike atmosphere'. On residential nurseries: 'It is undesirable for children in care to be brought up within the curtilage of a national assistance institution, even though the material conditions may be satisfactory, which is seldom the case.'[18] Apart from encouraging local authorities to improve their existing residential accommodation, the Home Office pressed for family group homes in place of large homes and cottage homes, they discouraged the use of residential nurseries, and encouraged the use of fostering, particularly for young children, as much as possible. The choice of the small, family group home was based on an assumption that it is possible to create within an environment which closely resembles family life and that children can be brought up in such a setting in much the same way as others living with their own families in the neighbourhood. Local authorities accepted the Home Office line and put their resources to establishing these small homes. A survey conducted in 1955 amongst 17 local authorities showed that of the 101 family group homes, 85 had been opened since 1950.

It also indicated some of the problems associated with this change of policy, for instance in staffing. The Home Office was training women as houseparents; the common practice in family group homes was to employ a married couple, who, more often than not, had no training and little or no experience of the problems of deprived children and the particular problems associated with personal relationships in a small human group; but the survey concluded on an optimistic note: 'If the limitations of an artificial family are accepted by all, if the members of the family are carefully selected and the staff of the right calibre, then the family group home can be one of the happiest forms of child care'.[19]

The general disapproval of the use of residential nurseries had been communicated to local authorities by the Home Office in 1950. In a memorandum of that year the Home Office advocated boarding-out or placement in a family group home as generally preferable to residential nursery care for the under-fives. The policy was underlined by Dr Bowlby's studies and others which pointed to the potential damage to young children of an upbringing in the often emotionally sterile surroundings of residential nurseries at a time in their lives when they most needed personal and continuous attention.[20] It was this evidence as much as the expense of nursery care, that led local authorities to avoid using them more than they could help. Some managed to close their nurseries altogether. Northumberland County Council made a special appointment in 1953 of a child care officer who was given the assignment of placing the 22 children in their residential nursery into foster homes or returning them to their parents; this proved successful and the nursery was closed.[21] The Eighth Children's Department Report of the Home Office noted approvingly the reduction in the number of nurseries to 166 on 31 December 1960 compared with 215 in November 1954 and the decrease of the number of children in them from 4,812 in 1954 to 3,543 in 1960, or 40% and 30% respectively of all children in care under the age of five.[22] This decrease continued to just under 20% in 1968.

There was an increase in the provision of hostels for working boys and girls. The number rose from 16 in 1949 to nearly 60 in 1954; this figure then remained virtually unchanged for the next six years, but had risen to 92 by 1966. Hostels tended to be used more for children who came into care later, often committed to care by the courts. Many of these young people presented serious behaviour problems and required particularly careful handling; but the staff capable of providing this was in short supply.

The problem of finding suitable accommodation for children coming into care was general; it was especially acute in relation to physically and mentally handicapped children and young offenders. This last group often exhibited social maladjustment which led to their committal by the courts. In 1952, about 2,000 children, about 4% of the total in care, were severely enough handicapped to need accommodation in special boarding homes and schools. Children's departments had no special accommodation of their own to offer to these children and relied on the education and health services, but both of these were themselves desperately short of special facilities. Delinquent, educationally sub-normal children formed a group for whom it proved particularly difficult to find suitable placements and children's departments considered this problem to be the most testing in the early fifties. It was the topic of a special meeting in 1953 between representatives of the local authority associations, the Ministry of Education and the Home Office. For some time the Association of Children's Officers had been pressing the Home Office to provide a number of special approved schools for these children, but the Home Office were reluctant to separate delinquent and non-delinquent educationally retarded children, whose needs were similar and amenable to being solved within the education service. So far as the delinquent part of this population was concerned, more encouragement could be given to the courts to commit such children to the care of the local authority, who could then send them to the special schools within the education system.

There is some evidence that juvenile courts did commit more educationally sub-normal and maladjusted children to care after these discussions, as a likely way of securing them special treatment. Children's departments might always be able to exert that extra bit of pressure to obtain the necessary places. This practice was later commented on with some disapproval by the Ingleby Committee which considered that the use of court proceedings to secure priority of special treatment was open to strong objection.[23]

The Home Office circulated a memorandum on Handicapped Children in Local Authority Care in 1954 which made some general suggestions on how children's departments might themselves try to absorb their own problems and pointed out the kind of help that could be obtained from local education, health and welfare authorities which had statutory functions. Lack of knowledge about where to seek help was however not the main problem, rather how to cause that help to materialize, for throughout the existence of the children's departments special facilities for handicapped children, in particular educationally sub-normal and maladjusted children, have always been in short supply.

By the late sixties the proportion of handicapped children in special accommodation to the total numbers in care had declined to a little over 3%. While one cannot rule out the possibility that lesser numbers of handicapped children were coming into care, it may also be suggested that children's departments were becoming more successful in absorbing them within their own, more diversified, accommodation, thus making it less necessary to seek specialized placements elsewhere.

Foster care

The Home Office exerted great efforts in the direction of fostering. The proportion of children in foster homes was shown right from the commencement as a separate item for each local authority in the annual abstract of statistics of children in care, and a kind of league table came into existence whereby local authorities which were successful in this respect would be held up as exemplary, a spur to greater effort on the part of the laggard ones. Foster care was considered (after adoption) as the next best substitute to a normal home life. There was in fact, little, if any, empirical evidence from this country available in the 1950s to support this belief.[24] The first Home Office Children's Department Report to be published following the implementation of the Children Act showed which local authority was the most and which the least successful in placing children in foster homes. The next two reports for the fifties, however, did not continue this rather embarrassing singling-out process. In fairness to the Home Office, it had no option but to press hard for a policy of fostering since this had been laid upon local authorities as a major duty under the Children Act.

Foster care was among the matters enquired into by a House of Commons Select Committee in 1951-2.[25] Their comments on it were a replica of comments made by the Home Office, the Curtis Committee and the earlier Poor Law committees that had considered the same matter. The Select Committee recognized that a policy of wholesale fostering was not to be pursued; there were qualifying considerations to be borne in mind which made it essential to weigh up each case individually. 'Neither boarding-out nor anything else connected with child care is either susceptible of wholesale treatment or to be regarded merely as an affair of theories and percentages', they said. Nonetheless, the Committee were impressed by the arguments in favour of fostering, and noted that it was also the cheapest form of care. In order to avoid any possibility of foster parents making a profit out of keeping foster children, the Home Secretary, had, in 1950, restricted local authorities to paying no more than £2 on average per child per week. In 1952, the average weekly cash fostering rate was actually only £1·44 per week as compared with the cost of £5·25 in a local authority home. Happily for the Exchequer and local authorities, if not necessarily for foster children or foster parents, the select committee noted that the figures revealed 'the striking and unusual fact that what is generally agreed to be the best method of providing for children in the care of local authorities is also the cheapest' and continued: 'it also points the way towards possible major economies which, far from endangering the fulfilment of the policy laid down by Parliament, would actually promote it'.

The Social Survey enquiry had revealed that two-thirds of the suggestions made by foster parents whom they questioned were concerned with improvements in allowances. The question posed was to what extent the limitation of allowances acted as a barrier to the expansion of fostering. The level of allowances had to be reconciled with the Home Office policy that foster parents should not make a profit out of their work. Probably most local authorities accepted the no-profit argument, but they must have found the £2 average per week per child limit an unnecessary restriction. Even in the mid-fifties, they were beginning to increase payment rates to people prepared to look after special cases, such as babies and enuretic, retarded or otherwise handicapped children. Some also introduced special schemes, paying a retaining fee to foster parents prepared to act as a stand-by for emergency cases; but until 1958, when the Local Government Act abolished the £2 limit, any payments above the average had to be balanced by payment below the average to others.

The expansion of fostering made slow but steady progress from 1949 onward. In that year 35% of all children in care were fostered. From then on, the percentage figure rose year by year until it reached 48% in 1960. Much of the expansion was no doubt due to the increased use of foster homes for very young children coming into care for short-term periods, and the determined efforts made to get babies out of nurseries. At the same time, children's departments ran foster homes recruitment campaigns for all age groups, and worked hard to get people interested in this form of ancillary social work.

Changes in residential care

Increasing numbers of children who have come to the attention of children's departments have kept up the pressure on accommodation of all types, and the departments have been hard pressed to meet the demand. Walton has accused the local authorities of maintaining insufficient residential care places, and thus being unable to cope with periods of extra pressure. He suggests that the use by local authorities of voluntary organizations' accommodation acts as a kind of barometer of this pressure. He also describes the voluntary organizations' work in this respect as having a 'safety valve function'.[26] In the early fifties one child out of every ten in care was sent to a voluntary home. The proportion dropped to 5·7% in 1963, but rose again to 6·4% in 1965 and 7·4% in 1968.

Pressure on residential accommodation resulted in part from the slowing down of the use of foster home placements. It has already been noted that the proportion of children in foster homes to the total number in care rose steadily from 1949 to 1960. This rise continued, to reach a peak of 52·2% in 1964. After that there was a slight drop in the figure every year and in 1968 it stood at 49·5%. The annual statistics do not, however, take account of the number of times a foster home may be used for different children in the course of a year, and short-term fostering is much used for the many children who come into care for brief periods. All the same there appears to have been a reaction against the earlier belief that every child could benefit from foster care and the research work carried out by Trasler and Parker[27] has been influential in stemming the tide of indiscriminate boarding-out. The Home Office in its report for 1961-3 had already conceded that fostering was not necessarily the best form of care for every child; that apart from those cases where it was ruled out on account of a child's physical or mental handicap, there were others where children, because of temperament or previous experience, could be more happily and successfully cared for in a children's home.[28] In terms of financial costs, fostering has remained the cheapest form of care. In 1968, the average cost for a child in a foster home was £3·21 per week compared with £14·27 for a child in a local authority home. Residential care had in fact begun to come into its own more as a positive form of care rather than a second best to fostering. In spite of the pressures brought about by the sheer increase in numbers, there have been some interesting changes in the forms of residential care in the past few years. The process of replacing out of date and unsuitable establishments has continued. In 1966 there were 1,577 homes of various sorts but only 352 had been used as children's homes before 1948. The use of nurseries also declined further despite a rise in the number of children under school age received into care. The policy of developing small group care units continued, either in purpose-built accommodation or in larger ones adapted for small group living. It is of interest to note that the use of the term 'family' group was gradually being abandoned in favour of 'small' group, as doubts were being expressed about the validity of the family model for group care of biologically un-related children and staff.[29] New ways of using residential care were also being developed, e.g. with residential staff working 'out' from the home with families of the children in their charge. In one local authority, Geoffrey Banner was experimenting with the integration of parents in the residential care programme, on the lines which had been developed in nurseries where, for instance, parents were encouraged to come in and put their young children to bed. He suggests that this kind of parent-participation can be utilized for older children, 'helping to get the tea, sitting down to a meal together, perhaps coming to stay for weekends or even, in the case of mothers in prisons, coming on a parole period of leave'.[30]

The provision of an increased number of small units has enabled many local authorities to create specialized accommodation to meet individual needs. Systematically gathered information on this is hard to come by, but examples can be quoted from some sources. The Home

Office reports of 1961-3 and 1964-6, tell of special provisions by some local authorities for children of disturbed mentality or from particularly difficult backgrounds. Tilley reports on the types of residential accommodation provided by Southampton children's department, which includes a home for emotionally disturbed children, and a home for boys who are admitted just prior to or early in adolescence. White describes the accommodation provided by the Lancashire children's department, which includes amongst its sixty-seven establishments a day centre, and a mother and baby home catering for a small number of difficult girls in care and their babies.[31] Sheffield children's department has developed a children's centre for between forty and fifty children to provide, on the one hand, an assessment and observation centre and on the other hand, a remedial long-term centre for children with behaviour disturbances.[32]

These are just a few instances of the kinds of development that have been taking place. They indicate a sensitive awareness of individual problems and a desire to meet these through specialized treatment facilities. Developments of this kind have helped to transform the image of residential care from a backwater to a service that is alive and ready to tackle special problems.

Adoption work

Although a great deal of adoption work had been and remained with the sixty-five or so voluntary adoption agencies, children's departments came into the picture immediately they had been set up in 1948. The Curtis Committee recommended that all children placed for adoption with persons other than their own parents should be supervised, and the Adoption Act 1950 placed this responsibility with local authorities, to be discharged through the child care service. In addition children's departments were to share in the work of guardian *ad litem* on behalf of those courts that were authorized to make adoption orders. The Children Act 1948 had also empowered local authorities to place children already in their care with adopters and from the mid-fifties onward this became quite a normal procedure; for example, 1,118 children were dealt with in this way in 1956, and 1,278 in 1960. These comprised about 3% of all annual discharges from care. In most cases the children so placed were illegitimate, with little prospect of eventual return to their own mothers.

Thus arranging adoptions for children already in care, supervision of children placed for adoption by other agencies and guardian *ad litem* work in respect of more than 80% of those awaiting adoption, formed an important part of children's departments' functions by the end of the fifties.

In order to minimize the risk attending privately arranged adoptions, the Hurst Committee[33] in 1954 had recommended that local authorities should be given power to act themselves as adoption agencies and this was granted in the Adoption Act of 1958. From the early sixties, an increasing number of them have done so. In 1966 there were 67, in 1967, 78 and in 1968 the number had reached 84 out of a possible 174 local authorities. The number of adoptions which resulted from placement through the agency of local authorities rose from about 3,000 annually in the earlier years to 3,600 in 1968. In many cases local authorities decided to set up their own adoption agencies so as to discourage direct and third party placements, although such privately arranged adoption arrangements are still legal, but there is some evidence that local authorities were being encouraged by the Home Office to involve themselves more in adoption placement work, probably more in those areas of the county where voluntary adoption agencies were sparsely represented.[34]

Child protection

Another area of work in which there was a notable expansion over the years was child protection. The recent legislation which governs local authorities' functions in this field stems, in the main, from the Children Act 1958, although child protection legislation dates back to 1872, when an Act was brought in to suppress the abuses of baby farming and to bring those foster parents who took children privately and often on a commercial basis, under public supervision and control. In the fifties, children's departments were supervising between 6,000 and 7,000 such children. Most of them lived with private foster parents, but some lived in private nurseries and other such establishments. After 1963 there came a steady increase in the number of cases for supervision. In 1968 it had reached 10,634, or 36% more than in 1958. This increase coincided with the growing influx of Commonwealth citizens, and the Home Office considered that the increase in private fostering was due in large part to the number of overseas students who had to find foster homes for their young children, yet whose circumstances were such that the latter could not be received into local authority care.[35]

The majority of children under supervision in private foster homes are concentrated around London and the adjoining counties. The total numbers are not large—about one-sixth of the numbers in care: but the growth in this area of care has made its contribution to the overall increase in the work of the departments.

Approved school after-care

Children's departments were drawn more and more into work with children in approved schools, a trend which also seems to date from the early sixties. The approved schools were organized as a separate service working under the guidance of the Home Office though some were actually provided by the local authorities. The connection between the approved school population and children in care was often quite a close one—some of those committed to the schools had been in care themselves or had a brother or sister in care. By the terms of the approved school order, a boy or girl released from the school had to undergo a period of supervision. In the early forties much of this work for boys had been carried out by Home Office appointed after-care agents who formed a small service largely separated from the mainstreams of social work. The Ingleby Committee, reviewing the after-care service, considered that it should cease to exist as a separate offshoot largely because the personnel were untrained, had to cover wide areas of the country and were forced to work in isolation from other social services. They recommended that the work should be shared in future between probation and children's departments. Subsequently the Children and Young Persons Act 1963 laid a duty on local authorities to act as after-care agents when asked by an approved school to do so. The children's departments were already empowered to undertake this work before 1963 but in view of the availability of an after-care service run direct by the Home Office, they never took on more than a small share of the work. After 1963, their share increased. In 1962 they had supervised 15% of the boys and 25% of the girls; by 1965, the most recent year for which figures are readily available, the proportions had increased to 37·7% and 25% respectively, probation officers being responsible for most of the remainder. In 1963 too, under the same Act, local authority children's departments were given the power to visit and befriend children who were in care at the time of their committal to a school, and many departments made use of that power. By 1968, 7,719 children were in contact with child care officers in one or other of these two ways, compared with 2,331 in 1962. While these duties are not as onerous and time-consuming as some others relating to children in care, this is another way in which the overall extent of work has grown up.

Notes

1. J. Wareham, *op. cit.,* p. 130.
2. *Sixth Report on the Work of the Home Office Children's Department,* H.M.S.O., 1951, p. 6
3. *The Family After 21 Years,* Lancs. C.C. Children's Department, 1968.
4. *The First Seven Years—Reflections on the Work of the Cheshire County Council Children's Committee, 1947-1954.*
5. *Then and Now, op. cit.,* p. 11.
6. *The First Four Years—Report of the Children's Officer of the City of Birmingham, 1949-1953,* p. 8.
7. *Eighth Report on the Work of the Home Office Children's Department,* H.M.S.O., 1961, p. 2.
8. J. Packman, *Child Care Needs and Numbers,* Allan & Unwin, 1968. Dr Packman's valuable study set out to establish the connections between numbers of children in care of various authorities and the factors that might contribute to the variations. In so far as she was able to generalize she suggested that social

conditions associated with high mobility might be powerful need-producing factors. Care proportions tended to be higher in the south and east than north and west and were generally larger in towns than counties. The availability of preventive and alternative care services in an area was also probably an important variable.

9. P. G. Gray and E. Parr, *Children in Care and the Recruitment of Foster Parents*, Social Survey 249, 1957.

10. In the Social Survey Study it was found that children in care because of parental illness stayed only a short time in care, while those in care because of illegitimacy, homelessness, parental death or desertion or through committal to care, tend to stay for a long time. These latter categories are those which make rehabilitation work particularly difficult and protracted.

11. R. Walton, 'The Development of the Residential Care of Deprived Children', *Child Care Quarterly Review*, Vol. 23, No. 3, July 1969, pp. 89-98.

12. *Home Office Report on the Work of the Children's Department 1964-1966*, p. 7.

13. Home Office—E. Grey, *Workloads in Children's Departments*, H.M.S.O., 1969, p. 22.

14. *Home Office Eighth Report*, pp. 2-3.

15. Home Office Circular No. 160/1948.

16. J. Bowlby, *Maternal Care and Mental Health*, W.H.O., 1951.

17. A.C.O. Bulletin, No. 35, December 1954.

18. *Home Office Sixth Report*, pp. 17-19.

19. A.C.O. Bulletin, No. 43, September 1955.

20. R. Dinnage and M. L. Kellmer Pringle, *Residential Child Care Facts and Fallacies*, National Bureau for Co-operation in Child Care and Longmans, 1967. The authors confirmed the earlier findings and conclude their remarks by stating that despite better staffing and more understanding attitudes there is little to shake and much to confirm accepted opinions that residential nurseries, apart from the earliest months of life and the shortest stay, should be a last resort for babies and young children.

21. J. Balls, *Where Love Is*, Gollancz, 1958.

22. *Home Office Eighth Report*, p. 12.

23. *Committee on Children and Young Persons* (Ingleby), Cmnd. 1191, H.M.S.O., 1960, para. 312.

24. Most of the evidence about fostering has since come to light in the sixties. There is a great deal of fostering breakdown which does not show up in published Home Office statistics. For a summary of the research see: R. Dinnage and M. L. Kellmer

Pringle, *Foster Home Care—Facts and Fallacies*, National Bureau for Co-operation in Child Care and Longmans, 1967.

25. *Sixth Report from the Select Committee on Estimates*, Session 1951-1952.

26. Walton, *op. cit.*, p. 98.

27. See G. B. Trasler, *In Place of Parents*, Routledge & Kegan Paul, 1960, and R. A. Parker, *Decision in Child Care*, Allen & Unwin, 1966.

28. Home Office Report 1961-1963, p. 4.

29. See J. Hodder, 'Management of Children's Department Residential Services', in *Residential Staff in Child Care*, R.C.C.A., Vol. 16, 1968.

30. G. A. Banner, 'Co-operation in Residential Care', in *Caring for Children*, ed. M. L. Kellmer Pringle National Bureau for Co-operation in Child Care, 1969, pp. 86-95.

31. See papers presented by T. White and F. Roger Tilley to the Cropwood Round-Table Conference. Published in *Community Homes and the Approved School System*, University of Cambridge, Institute of Criminology, 1969.

32. *Nineteenth Annual Report of the Work of the Children's Department of the City of Sheffield*, 1968, p. 7.

33. *Report of the Departmental Committee on the Adoption of Children, 1954* (Hurst Report), H.M.S.O., Cmnd. 9248.

34. Child Adoption No. 53, 1968, p. 53.

35. Supporting evidence comes from Dr Packman's study, *op. cit.*, p. 132, f.n. This gives a correlation coefficient of 0.56 for the relationship between the number of children in private placements (triennial average 1957-59) and the proportion of the population born outside England and Wales, for 53 industrial towns.

4

Policy developments — the Children and Young Persons Act 1963

The child neglected in his own home

At about the time that the new child care service was set up, the situation of the child neglected in his own home came up for debate and aroused public concern. The Curtis Committee, very much alive to the problem, had taken the view that it did not come within their terms of reference, and could only urge that it should be given attention elsewhere. Soon after the Committee had reported, a privately sponsored report came out which focused on children deprived of a normal upbringing, though living with their own parents. The report was the work of the Women's Group on Public Welfare,[1] the same group that had produced 'Our Towns—A Close Up' a few years earlier. The authors saw their report as a sequel-cum-preface to the work of the Curtis Committee, a sequel because it came out later, and a preface because it broke off where the latter had begun. Their concern with the neglected child living in his own home arose from the fact that, despite the prevalence of such neglect, little attention was being given to the problem. In one year alone, 1944-5, the N.S.P.C.C. had dealt with more than 107,000 children coming from 41,000 different families. The number of people found guilty of cruelty against children in the period 1940-4 was the highest since the period 1925-9 and the figure for 1945, 1,769, was higher than for any five year period during the past twenty years. Although these figures did not necessarily represent absolute increases in child neglect (they only reflected the increase of *successful prosecutions* and had not been related to changes in the child population over the period), nevertheless, they added weight to the proposition that the problem of child cruelty and neglect was substantial. In addition, the group cited evidence from the cases which came to the notice of child care agencies, both statutory and voluntary, which pointed to a considerable number of children coming into care because of neglect situations within their family setting.

The report was published at a time when the subject of the 'problem family' was very much under discussion. A series of publications, many of them the results of local surveys, indicated that there were in the community a small proportion of families whose ability to cope with the society's standards of child rearing was at an unacceptably low level.[2] There had already been some discussion in social work and public health circles about what could be done to get at the causes, if possible, and to raise the standards of social functioning in such families. The specific problem of child neglect fitted into these discussions since it featured in the publications on problem families.

Two short debates on child neglect in Parliament during July and December 1949 led to a Government promise of investigation. Coming so soon after the Curtis report and the Monckton enquiry it must have been a matter of some slight embarrassment to Whitehall to see yet another stone uncovered to reveal a state of affairs which really should have formed a part of the Curtis Committee's enquiries.

In the event a working party from the Home Office, the Ministry of Health and the Ministry of Education made an examination of the situation and reported to their respective ministers. The conclusion reached was that no extension of statutory powers was required, nor was there a need for a departmental committee of enquiry. What was required was the better co-ordination of the available local authority and other statutory services together with the resources of the voluntary agencies. This was the gist of the statement which the Home Secretary made to the House of Commons in July 1950.[3] The statement was followed by a joint ministerial circular addressed to local authorities advising them on the kind of action they might take in connection with the discovery of child neglect and child cruelty in their area.[4]

The co-ordination issue

The advice contained in the joint circular was mainly concerned with the establishment of the machinery for co-ordination at local level. The circular pointed out that local authorities, in their capacities as authorities for education, welfare, health, housing and child care, already had the necessary powers to assist families and thus avoid the enforced removal of children from their homes. Where financial aid was needed, then the National Assistance Board might be able to assist. There were many voluntary organizations specially formed to deal with child neglect and cruelty. Thus far, the circular made the point which had already been made in Parliament, that the means and the powers were already there to bring the problem under control. There then followed specific suggestions for forming co-ordination committees or designating an officer to be responsible for initiating co-ordination; in either case regular meetings of officers of the local authority and other statutory services and representatives of voluntary organizations should be planned, and a designated officer should be notified of cases of child neglect and ill-treatment so that coherent action could be taken.

Local authority response to the recommendation to establish co-ordinating machinery was considered by the Home Office to have been good. The *Seventh Home Office Children's Department Report*, 1955, noted that 123 authorities had designated a co-ordinating officer, in nearly half of them the children's officer. Coverage however was hardly uniform. For example, a study by Donnison, published in 1954, showed that while in Salford machinery had been set up for co-ordinating social work, none existed in neighbouring Manchester.[5] And from the evidence submitted in the mid-fifties to the Younghusband Committee only about two-thirds of responding authorities said they were generally satisfied with the arrangements that had been made. One fault lay in the tendency to deal with families that had already got past the prevention stage; thus there was a tendency to depart from the original purpose behind the co-ordination concept which was to get on the scene early. But there were other, deeper-lying reasons which militated against successful co-ordinated effort. They have been analysed by Julia Parker under three headings: the need for early referral, the common agreement required about the action needed in each case, and probably the most important of the three, the availability of social workers with the time and skill to carry out the committee's decisions. Mrs Parker suggests that this last factor arose from a lack of recognition of social work as a profession with its own skills. Health visitors, nurses and education welfare officers were reluctant to entrust work to child care officers unless they could be sure that they had specific skills which they themselves did not possess.[6]

Evidence collected in the mid-sixties for the Committee on the Management of Local Government confirmed the difficulties encountered in the translation of co-ordination theory into practice. It seems that co-ordination often got bogged down in interminable discussion of cases without the necessary action following, and departmental rivalries acted as blocks to progress. Co-ordination by committees of senior officers tended to be as often inhibiting as enabling; but where co-ordination at field level was encouraged, successful handling of families was likely to ensue.[7]

However chequered the development of co-ordination, the circular and subsequent administrative action focused attention on the issue of preventive work, and paved the way to specific statutory authority for it. It is difficult to measure the effect of co-ordination. The N.S.P.C.C. figures of cases dealt with declined from 40,198 in 1949-50 to 38,326 in 1959-60; but the decline may have been partially due to the fact that the local authorities were moving more and more into this traditional N.S.P.C.C. field. No national statistics on this facet of local authority work are available.

Co-ordination formed one of the topics discussed by the Ingleby Committee. It arose out of their general discussion on the means for providing support through the social services to families whose children were 'at risk', who might be prevented from coming before juvenile court or received into care. In the mid-fifties, the government had its attention drawn to the work of the juvenile courts and the means at their disposal for dealing with young offenders. The last review of these issues had been undertaken in 1927 by a Departmental Committee on Young Offenders. Now the Magistrates' Association suggested that the time was ripe for a fresh review. It seemed feasible to combine an enquiry into juvenile delinquency with a more general enquiry into the working of those social services concerned with the family, since there was evidence that juvenile delinquency and child neglect were rooted in the same causes. The government accepted the need for an enquiry, and on 3 October 1956 appointed a Departmental Committee under the chairmanship of Viscount Ingleby. The committee, known as the Committee on Children and Young Persons, reported in October 1960.

The Ingleby Report

The main preoccupation of the Ingleby Committee was with the theme of prevention: the prevention of juvenile delinquency and child neglect and, to a lesser extent, of the reception of children into care for all manner of reasons. Juvenile delinquency figures in particular had risen steeply in the post-war years. They reached a peak in 1951, then started to drop slightly before soaring upwards again. It had been considered that the rise in the immediate post-war years could be attributed to the disruptions caused by the war: evacuation, air-raids and the absence of father from home. Once the young wartime generation had grown up, it was argued, things would improve; but by 1958, it was clear that this was not the case. There was a great increase in crime in the population generally, both in the number and the seriousness of offences, and this was particularly serious in the age-group 14 to 21. As the Ingleby Committee pointed

68

out, the position fifteen years after the end of the war, far from improving, was more serious than it had ever been.

The Ingleby Committee were not asked to conduct a detailed enquiry into the causes of juvenile delinquency, but they took as a basic premise the view that the root of the problems of both delinquency and child neglect lay in the quality of family life. From that, they argued, it followed that it was the duty of the State to do what it could to aid the family so that it might function adequately. 'Everything within reason must be done to ensure that children are not neglected but that they get the best upbringing possible', they commented, and while they held to the fundamental belief that the primary responsibility for bringing up children was parental, it was 'the duty of the community to provide through its social and welfare services the advice and support which such parents and children need; to build up their capacity for responsibility and to enable them to fulfil their proper role'.[8] The suggestion that the State's services should be involved only when the family is seen to be failing in its parental role was emphasized a number of times throughout the report. They stressed the responsibility of parents in bringing up their children, and the responsibility of young persons for their own behaviour in society. Unfortunately we cannot here take the discussion further into that interesting field, for we must confine ourselves to the aspects of prevention in the committee's recommendations. In pursuing this particular theme, they undertook a somewhat cursory review of those community social services which already existed to help families.[9] They began by mentioning the functions of the Children Act 1948 and noted the Home Office circular of that year which pointed to the desirability of preventing reception into care wherever possible, but observed that local authorities had no statutory authority for undertaking this work. They referred to the various functions of the National Health Service Act 1946, and discussed the duties and powers of local health authorities relating to the care of expectant and nursing mothers and of pre-school children; the arrangements which could be made for the general prevention of illness: the provision of health visitors, home nurses and home-helps; day nurseries, and the care and after-care of mentally disordered people. They also commented on the recently passed Mental Health Act 1959 and the facilities which the local authority would have to provide: residential accommodation, occupation and training centres, and social clubs—a full range of services, including those of trained social workers, which would cater for the mentally disordered who did not require hospital and specialist treatment.

They went on to note the duties of the local welfare authorities under the National Assistance Act 1948 to provide residential accommodation for the aged and infirm, the blind, deaf or dumb and for handicapped children; and they mentioned the facilities of the (then) National Assistance Board to provide financial assistance. Local authority health and welfare functions were also referred to—the school health services, meals in schools and provision of clothing to enable children to attend school. Housing services under the Housing Acts received a mention, specifically the local housing authorities' duties of examining houses as to their fitness for human habitation, the abatement of overcrowding, and the provision of accommodation. A brief reference to the part played by the probation service concluded the survey of statutory services, but the work of some voluntary organizations was also mentioned, for instance the N.S.P.C.C., Family Service Units, the Family Welfare Association, the W.V.S. and the Salvation Army, all providing family support.

The picture of the services, particularly the statutory services, so presented was quite an impressive one—on paper at least—but nowhere in the report was any doubt cast on their ready availability to the public or the capacity of any service theoretically available to do the job it was created to do. There is a certain naïvety of thinking in this part of the report; but the committee did at least make the point that the public should be informed of the various services, including those of voluntary organizations, which were available to help in time of need and should be told where to apply for advice.

The committee seemed to think that the main need was for better co-ordination between the services, citing the Home Office circular of 1950 as an example of what they wished to see more widely achieved. They tried to be helpful by putting forward an analysis of the three stages which they distinguished in dealing with the prevention of neglect in the home:

1. Detection of families at risk.
2. Investigation and diagnosis of the particular problem.
3. Treatment—the provision of facilities and services to meet the needs of families and to reduce the stresses and dangers that they face.

At the first stage—detecting families at risk—the committee thought the responsibility should be spread over the widest possible front. Many people should be involved: neighbours, teachers, medical practitioners, ministers of religion, health visitors, district nurses and so on—anyone who learned at first hand of a family which might be in trouble. The second stage—investigation and diagnosis —might be undertaken by a unit within the local authority where skilled and concentrated attention could be given to a case. In the larger local authorities this might be done by a family advice centre or family bureau which would serve as a central reference point both for the various local authority services and for members of the public.

The third stage, treatment, should remain in the hands of existing agencies, both statutory and voluntary, and should be decided upon in consultation with the various departments likely to be concerned. This is where the Ingleby Committee's advocacy of good co-ordination was focused. They also considered that in the larger local authorities, responsibility for co-ordination should be in the hands of a family advice centre, independent of departmental loyalties, and headed by a senior officer with direct access to the clerk of the authority rather than to a committee.

The committee received evidence from a number of social work organizations which expressed the view that for effective preventive work a skilled, intensive casework service was required and that local authorities should have power to give material aid where necessary. Some claimed that the children's department should be given this task, on the grounds that the prevention of neglect, the provision of alternative forms of care and the restoration of a child to his family were all parts of what was basically one operation. Others thought that this work should be given to the health department and pointed to the importance of the role of the health visitor. There were also suggestions by some witnesses that a new local authority department should be created out of the existing children's departments and those parts of the health department's work concerned with preventive functions.

Faced with this conflicting evidence on organizational structures, the committee commented that the long-term solution might possibly lie in a reorganization of the various services concerned with the family to form a unified family service.[10] They became thus the first official body publicly to voice a view which was to reach its full expression in the Seebohm Report of 1968.

In the meantime they had somehow to deal with the existing structure. They saw the solution as lying in the improvement of co-ordination on the basis of the three-fold division of functions. In order to ensure maximum flexibility and an adequacy of power, they recommended that a general duty should be laid upon local authorities to prevent or forestall the suffering of children through neglect in their own homes. To make this effective, local authorities should provide preventive casework services, and meet material needs that could not be met from other sources.

They did not grasp the nettle of deciding which local authority department should be given this function, but recommended that it should be vested generally in the local authority.

On the preventive side the Ingleby Committee had not come up with any startling innovations. Their survey of existing personal social services convinced them that these were sufficient in scope to support badly-functioning families, if only those responsible for running these services could get together and co-ordinate their work. Nonetheless some minor changes could be made, including the enactment of specific statutory authority for undertaking preventive work, so as to put that particular issue beyond legal doubt.

The 1963 Act

The Ingleby proposals were incorporated in a Children and Young Persons Bill which received its Second Reading in the House of Lords in November 1962.[11] The first clause of the Bill dealt with the preventive work proposals. It received a unanimous welcome from both sides of the House, every peer who spoke on it seeing it as a sensible and logical provision. The issue of which local authority department should be asked to undertake the work was resolved when the Minister of State at the Home Office, Earl Jellicoe, told the House of the Government view that the new duties and powers were such a natural extension of the existing ones of children's committees that they should also be exercised by them.[12]

The Bill passed into law, and Section 1 of the Children and Young Persons Act 1963 came into operation on 1 October of that year. This placed a duty on county and county borough councils to make available such advice, guidance and assistance as might promote the welfare of children by diminishing the need to receive them into care, keep them in care, or to bring them before a court. It also provided for assistance to be given in kind or in cash to this end. The authority for the work was limited to cases where there was a genuine risk of children having to be received into care or to appear before court, but action could also be taken in situations which might lead to the return home of children already in care.[13] To this extent the section was limited. Childless

74

families, however great their problems, were excluded, as were families whose children could not justifiably be said to be 'at risk', though no doubt in practice the imagination could always be stretched to include a particular case in the 'at risk' category.

A Home Office circular explaining the new duties was addressed to local authorities shortly before the Act became operational.[14] This stressed the existence of statutory and voluntary agencies on which children's departments might draw to assist them in their preventive work. It emphasized that they were not to usurp work that was already being undertaken by other departments and voluntary organizations, but to fill any gaps which they might discover. The circular also referred to the new power to make cash payments to clients. It stressed that this should be exercised only in exceptional circumstances. Cash payments and welfare work had been kept separate in the post-war social welfare programme largely as the result of the rejection of Poor Law policies and as Professor Marshall has noted, the cash payment provision in Section 1 created a breach, albeit a minor one, in a policy which had operated for more than fifteen years.[15]

Effects on the service

Section 1 imposed potentially far-reaching functions on children's departments. It was explicit about these; but neither the Act nor Home Office Circulars made any mention of the extra resources necessary to carry them out. Nobody had a clear idea of the likely workload that would fall on local authorities and no official estimate of needs or numbers, or of the number of additional staff needed, both field and other, appears to have been made. An unofficial estimate however had appeared in 1961. In that year, in her address to the annual conference of the Association of Children's Officers, the Children's Officer of Oxfordshire, Mrs Barbara Kahan, brought together the known numbers of cases dealt with during 1959-60 by various statutory and voluntary agencies.[16] Children's departments had dealt with 42,000 receptions into care, and had nearly 62,000 children in care at the end of the period. Voluntary organizations were looking after a further 19,000; 112,000 children and young persons had been involved in complaints investigated and found substantiated by the N.S.P.C.C. and 52,000 had appeared before the courts and had been found guilty of indictable offences. 'Many thousands more,' she added, 'unfortunately unable to be counted at present were investigated by children's departments under the Children and Young Persons (Amendment) Act, 1952 or were referred to probation officers and health visitors. Taking into account the known figures and trying to make an intelligent guess at the unknown, it would appear that possibly at least 300,000 children and young persons under 18 were known to be in situations of actual or potential neglect in the broad sense during the year 1959-60.' Given that at that time there was a child population of approximately 12¼ millions under the age of eighteen in England and Wales, the estimate of 300,000 represented a figure of about 41 per thousand.

This constituted a substantial proportion likely to require attention, and of course, as Mrs Kahan pointed out, there was the unknown quantity, the 'dark' figure which was likely to emerge only as new statistics were collected and published. After the preventive section of the Act had become operational, the Home Office gathered additional information from local authorities on the number of children whose circumstances had been investigated and where need for reception into care had been averted by some positive action. The figure had grown from 31,140 children in 1964-5 to 161,339 (from 65,458 families) during 1967-8, not including cases which were still under investigation.

Under the Children and Young Persons Act 1963 local authorities are required to report to the Home Secretary not less than once in twelve months on the kind of provision they are making under Section 1. In 1964 the Home Office published a summary of reports. This did not reveal anything that was startlingly new, but it drew attention to some interesting developments. Increases in staff establishments had been approved by most local authorities and in some it had been possible to transfer field staff from other departments, usually Health Departments to Children's Departments. Co-operation with voluntary organizations and local charities had been strengthened. Nearly twenty authorities reported that the children's department had taken over, or expected to take over, responsibility for the temporary accommodation of homeless families or those in need of rehabilitation; and a number of children's departments were given responsibility for such families in various other ways, e.g. by undertaking social work with them in temporary accommodation or by liaising with housing departments over the allocation of permanent accommodation for them.

A substantial minority of authorities reported that they had decided to establish advice centres in response to the Ingleby Committee's recommendation that such a centre should be made available to which parents could turn for help and counsel. These centres might take different

forms: some would be units within the children's departments, others would be set up separately to service the
local agencies and others still would be located in a sub-
area to serve the local neighbourhood.[17]

Assistance in each case was used sparingly, most children's committees seemingly taking the view that every pre-
caution should be taken to avoid giving the impression
that the children's department was another National
Assistance Board.

The Home Office have not repeated the publication of
a summary report and apart from the annual reports
issued by some children's departments, which usually have
only a local distribution, the social work literature contains only occasional references to developments; but these
are taking place. Section 1 was drafted sufficiently widely
to allow for experimentation. Rent guarantee schemes,
half-way housing, and intensive work with selected families who have special difficulties in coping with their affairs,
are among the schemes that have been launched or extended.[18] One published report of innovation comes from
the London Borough of Brent which describes the use
made of residential housemothers who take over the care
of children at their own homes so as to avoid reception
into care, either living in if the accommodation is suitable
or coming in daily.[19] This use of housemothers who provide a 'care' element in their work is an extension of the
use of home-helps in similar situations.

The advent of Section 1 confirmed a shift in focus in
child care. The Children Act 1948 concentrated on meeting
the needs of the child in care; now the work moved to-
ward providing greater support for families with dependent
children in order to avert the need for care where possible.
This policy change began before 1963 but the legislation

of that year set the stamp of approval on it and as such the Act became an important landmark in the development of the child care service.

Notes

1. Women's Group on Public Welfare, *The Neglected Child and His Family*, O.U.P., 1948.

2. The report referred to nine publications by different medical officers of health on the subject of the 'problem family'; all were published between 1943 and 1947.

3. Nonetheless, an amendment to the Children and Young Persons Act was made in 1952, relating to the definition of child neglect and making it clear that children could be dealt with under care or protection provisions in cases where parents had not *wilfully* caused it.

4. *Joint Circular from the Home Office, Ministry of Health and Ministry of Education on Children Neglected or Ill-treated in their Own Homes*, 31 July 1950. Another circular issued by the Ministry of Health in 1954, pointed out the part which local authority health departments were empowered to play in dealing with family problems.

5. D. V. Donnison, *The Neglected Child and the Social Services*, Manchester University Press, 1954.

6. J. Parker, *op. cit.*, pp. 54-8.

7. *Management of Local Government*, Vol. 5, H.M.S.O., 1967, Ch. 12; see in particular pp. 353-8.

8. Ingleby Report, para. 8.

9. In point of fact the whole of the committee's discussion on child neglect and the need for preventive work with families occupied only 11 out of 179 pages of their report.

10. Ingleby Report, para. 47.

11. *Hansard*, Vol. 244, No. 10, 20 November 1962.

12. *Ibid.*, Col. 808.

13. See *Report on the Work of the Children's Department—Home Office, 1961-1963*. H.C. 155, p. 1.

14. Home Office Circular 204/1963.

15. T. H. Marshall, *Social Policy*, Hutchinson, 1965, p. 128.

16. B. J. Kahan, 'Prevention and Rehabilitation'. Reprint from *Approved Schools Gazette*, December 1961.

17. An exploratory study of a sample of sixteen advice centres

presents an optimistic picture of their future, concluding that they 'may very well become the wide, open door of our whole, big social service structure, acting as the "eyes and ears" of the social service system, helping us to see where the needs are and to hear what the people have to tell us'. See A. Leissner, *Family Advice Services*, Longmans, in association with National Bureau for Co-operation in Child Care, 1967.

There is also an interesting account of the setting-up of a Detached Advice Centre, which, amongst other things, resulted in a drop of receptions into care. For this see: D. Rumnicles, 'The Development of a Detached Family Advice Centre in a High Problem Area', *Case Conference*, Vol. 14, No. 7, November 1967, pp. 252-7.

18. See the *Bulletins of the Association of Children's Officers*, Nos. 113, January 1963, 120, March 1964, 124, December 1964.

19. H. Whalley, 'Children Into Care in their Own Homes', *British Hospital and Social Service Review*, Vol. LXXIX, No. 4113, 14 February 1969.

5

Policy developments — future trends

The call for a family service

The Ingleby report stimulated further discussion about the need for a family service. The committee had heard witnesses from a number of organizations which advocated such a service—urging the integration and simplification of personal social services to this end. In their evidence to the committee, the Council for Children's Welfare in association with the Fisher Group, had presented a cogent case.[1] They based their arguments on the premise that the family is a fundamental biological and social unit in the community, the living group in which children are brought up, yet, they pointed out, among all the wide and varied social services none existed to alleviate *family* stress, prevent breakdown and re-establish *family* life. The effect of the existing social service administrative arrangements had been to offer families a series of services, rigidly segregated and frequently duplicated. The two groups suggested a local authority family service which would help the 'well' family exposed to undue strain as well as providing early treatment for the 'sick' family, which might continue to function at some reasonably acceptable level with such help but without it would disintegrate. This service would also encompass the incomplete family, broken by desertion or by unmarried parenthood.

A similar proposal came from Professor Donnison in a Fabian publication.[2] Donnison's essay was published soon after Ingleby reported and he was afraid that the committee's recommendations might lead to the establishment of yet another local authority department concerned with personal social work. In his view there were already too many separate social work departments. 'The most urgent need ... is for the integration and simplification of existing services ... a new and separate service in yet another department of local government is precisely what is not wanted,' he wrote. As it turned out the advice was heeded, since the preventive service was allocated to an already existing department; but Donnison took the opportunity of arguing strongly for an examination of the whole array of personal services, not only those designed for deprived children but also the equally complex networks then developing to assist old people, the physically handicapped, the mentally disordered and so on, for whom the term 'community care' was being applied. He looked forward to the time when a service, and he too used the phrase *family service*, would be established in every area capable of providing facilities for a wide range of disadvantaged groups—from deprived children, people with marital problems, people in need of information about services, including the complexities of housing services and so on.

The expressions about the need for a *family* service had grown out of the dissatisfaction with the fragmentation of social services, particularly the personal social services. It is of interest to note that the criticisms rested on much the same rationale that had applied to the fragmentation of the administrative organization in the child care services at the time of the Curtis enquiry, only now they extended beyond this relatively narrow sphere into the wider personal services designed to meet the needs of adults as well as children. In essence the argument now was that services were administratively aimed at identifiable groups, e.g. the mentally disordered, the unmarried mother, the homeless etc. Any one official agency could have administrative responsibility for any one of these groups. Yet a number of social or physical handicaps could be concentrated in one family—or even more to the point—in one person, such as for example the mentally sub-normal, unmarried mother who was also homeless. Whose responsibility was she? This was the kind of situation about which questions were now being asked. The Ingleby committee had not deal with them—they were outside their terms of reference.

During the early sixties there were further calls for a family service. One of these came from a Labour Party study group under Lord Longford.[3] This foreshadowed what a Labour government might do in this field of social policy if elected to power. The Longford study group was mainly concerned with the problem of crime prevention by, among other measures, improvements in the social services. Like others who reviewed the administrative structure, they considered that it was 'ripe for review'. In their view, a new family service would incorporate and develop some of the functions of existing central and local government departments relating to children and families in general, including children's departments and parts of the health, welfare and education departments.

Their ideas were in fact very much in line with others who considered the time was due for the rationalization of the personal social services. In Scotland, the Kilbrandon committee, the Scottish equivalent of Ingleby, proposed a family-type service for that country and subsequently Scotland went ahead with its Social Work Act which became operative in November 1969.

For England and Wales, the Labour government, elected in October 1964, made a start by publishing a White Paper in the following year called: 'The Child, the Family and the Young Offender'.[4] It set out provisional proposals for practical reforms to support the family, to forestall and reduce delinquency and to revise the law and practice relating to offenders up to the age of 21. It was put forward as a discussion document. One of its more radical suggestions was the abolition of the juvenile court system in favour of non-judicial tribunals administered by local authorities. It is not the intention here to pursue the fate of that particular proposal which shocked some professionally interested groups such as magistrates and probation officers into instant opposition, except to say that it was withdrawn and the subject of trial procedures reintroduced in watered down and more conventional form in a further White Paper in 1968. We will return to this later in the chapter. But another, less controversial proposal in the 1965 White Paper was the appointment of a small independent committee to review the organization and responsibilities of the local authority personal social services and to consider what changes were desirable to ensure an effective family service. This proposal was very much linked with delinquency prevention. 'Preventive work with families, mainly undertaken in children's departments is of cardinal importance both for its positive social value and as a means of exposing situations which might give rise to delinquency' ran a passage in the White Paper. There was an echo of the Longford proposals in the proposal for a family service, drawing together functions from various existing departments.

The Seebohm report

The promised committee was swiftly set up in December 1965. Its chairman was Mr (now Sir Frederic) Seebohm, already known to social workers through his connection with the National Institute for Social Work Training. There was also a strong representation in the committee of people who had first hand social work experience. Their terms of reference were: 'to review the organisation and responsibilities of the local authority personal social services in England and Wales, and to consider what changes are desirable to secure an effective family service'. The report, published in July 1968,[5] proved to be a substantial one. The committee had no hesitation in condemning the way in which the services were organized. Fragmentation led to the duplication of some functions, gaps in the services and a tendency for departments to shift responsibility. They recommended a new local authority department, providing a community-based and family-orientated service which would be available to all, not only for families with children, and which would 'reaching far beyond the discovery and rescue of social casualties seek to involve the greatest number of individuals to act reciprocally, giving and receiving service for the well-being of the whole community'.

The new social services department would have responsibilities going beyond those of existing local authority departments, but would include:

(a) the present services provided by children's departments;
(b) welfare services provided under the National Assistance Act 1948;

(c) education, welfare and child guidance services;
(d) home-help services, mental health social work services, adult training centres, day nurseries and other social work services provided by health departments;
(e) certain social work currently undertaken by some housing departments.

We shall have to confine discussion of the Seebohm report to its effect on the child care service, but it should be said of the report generally that the proposals in it, as implemented, will in time change the nature and scope of social work, help the public to obtain a more effective service and give social workers a clearer sense of professional identity. And the establishment of the British Association of Social Workers in place of a number of separate professional organizations for social workers will give further impetus to the development of the profession.

To return to the likely effect of the Seebohm proposals on the child care service: the radical but quite logical suggestion of creating a new social service department at local authority level spells the end of children's committees and departments as constituted at present. Reorganization on these lines means that services to deprived children will become part of a wider-reaching service extending to the aged, the physically and mentally handicapped, the childless family, the single adult, the one-parent family: in fact to all age groups with a great variety of social needs. This is likely to produce a better organizational pattern for social work, but there is a possibility that some of the significant advances made in child care practice will be lost. The setting up of a specialized service in 1948 was undertaken precisely because a more generalized service had not met the needs of deprived children. It must be conceded here that this fear has not been expressed by commentators from the child care field who have published views on the Seebohm report. A joint statement by the respective presidents of the Association of Children's Officers and the Association of Child Care Officers welcomed the report as 'laying the foundations for a rational, imaginative and comprehensive service for people in need of social care' and went on to say that: 'the new social services department should have a clear responsibility for a wide range of social and personal problems'.[6] Another well-known writer on child care, Mrs Kahan, commented in similar vein: 'For child care workers there will be the encouragement of being able at least to look at the needs of children as a whole not just those deprived of family care and socially at risk but also the young offender, the handicapped, the school child in difficulties, the badly housed, fatherless families and the needs of the very young ... (it) is now likely to lead to a wider and more liberal social service for adults as well as children, a development which will owe much to the effects of twenty years of a unified child care service'.[7] No doubts were expressed about the possible loss of carefully built-up expertise, improved residential facilities and community goodwill; perhaps it was assumed that these achievements of the child care service could be maintained and extended in a wider service.

At the time of the publication of the Seebohm Report, the Government was awaiting the report of the Redcliffe-Maud Commission on Local Government. This was published in June 1969.[8] The Seebohm Committee had considered that their proposals should be implemented as soon as possible; in their view the need for swift action over-rode other considerations such as the adjustment of local government structures;[9] but there were other plans for reorganization, for example, in the health service, to be taken into consideration. The Government's view was expressed in the House of Lords debate on the Seebohm report by the Minister of State at the Home Office, Lord Stonham: 'Seebohm does not and cannot stand alone. It has to be considered in the context of the reorganization of the health service ... one must have regard to the proposals regarding the size and function of local authorities ...; from the Royal Commission on Local Government ... ; also relevant and already issued and under consideration is the Report on the Management of Local Government from which the Seebohm recommendations differ in a material respect'.[10] The report on the Management of Local Government had been published in 1967.[11] It strongly recommended a drastic reduction in the number of local authority committees in order to improve management efficiency and proposed that similar or related local government services should be grouped and allocated to one committee. This suggested a merger between children's departments and health and welfare departments, producing a different framework from that recommended in the Seebohm report. It did not commend itself to some professional social workers in the child care service, who were bitterly opposed to any suggestion of a straightforward merger with the local health services because of the fear that this would subsume social work under the Medical Officer of Health whose interest, it was generally believed by social workers, did not lie in that direction.[12] But in the meantime, some of the London boroughs, created in 1965 from the dissolution of the erstwhile London County Council, Middlesex and other local government areas around London, had been engaging in departmental amalgamations and their schemes included the setting up of single committees to deal with social services and health matters, contrary to the Seebohm proposals. This pre-empting did not meet with government approval.[13] It also met with strong disapproval from the Association of Child Care Officers which blacklisted some of the local authorities concerned.

The Local Authority Social Services Bill designed to give effect to the Seebohm proposals was introduced in the House of Commons and given an unopposed second reading on 26 February 1970. Not all the Seebohm Committee proposals required legislation for their implementation and the Bill was quite brief. It required local authorities to set up a social services committee and appoint a Director of Social Services together with adequate staff. The committee's functions would consist of those at present performed by children and welfare committees plus those services performed up to now by health committees which the Seebohm Committee had considered should be transferred to the new service (see page 86). But education welfare services were not being transferred and future responsibility for the administration of the child guidance service remained to be decided by the government. Of the other major function which was proposed for the new service by the Seebohm Committee, housing welfare, there was no mention in the Bill. In the main, however, the Bill followed predictably along the lines of the committee's proposals but while unification of personal social services at local level would be largely catered for, split ministerial responsibility remained, a point which was commented on in the debate on the second reading; a clause in the Bill stated that local authorities shall exercise their social service function under the guidance of the Secretary of State, i.e. the Home Secretary, but certain functions were explicitly excepted from this provision, namely those which relate to certain services for the aged and handicapped as well as to mothers and young children. Such services were already subject to some control by the Secretary of State for Health and Social Security and will continue under his guidance. On the other hand the opportunity was taken to unify social work training by the creation of a Central Council which may well operate independently of any ministry. A rationalization of social work training had become as necessary as the similar exercise on the social work side, since fragmentation of training tended to be equally wasteful of resources.

Because of the impending election, the later stages of the Bill were hurried through Parliament and the Bill received the Royal Assent on 29 May, the new, unified services being scheduled to commence operating from 1 April 1971.

'Children in Trouble' and the Children and Young Persons Act 1969

While the Seebohm campaign was being pursued, the child care service had to prepare to adjust itself to the plans which were put forward in the White Paper: 'Children in Trouble',[14] and published three months before the Seebohm report. This White Paper of 1968 was the successor to that of 1965 which had been quietly shelved. The revised proposals covered changes affecting the court procedures and post-court treatment of juveniles up to the age of seventeen. The reforms outlined were intended to be complementary to developments concerned with the prevention and treatment of juvenile delinquency and with other similar problems affecting children and their families, and would fit in with the Seebohm plans. Changes in legal procedures were suggested but, unlike the White Paper of 1965, the 1968 White Paper proposed the retention of the juvenile court system. Relatively little delay ensued in transforming the White Paper proposals into law. Although there was considerable debate in both Houses of Parliament on certain of the judicial issues involved, eighteen months after the proposals were first published, they became law substantially in their original form in the Children and Young Persons Act 1969. The Act provides for the substitution of non-criminal, care procedures in place of criminal procedures for the 'child' age group, i.e. the 10-14 years olds, and a more liberal use of the former instead of criminal procedures in the case of the 'young person' group, i.e. the 14-17 year age group. The White Paper had envisaged that in any case many juveniles would be dealt with under preventive action and therefore would not need to be brought before the court. Local authorities will also be drawn much more closely into work with young offenders, through having to maintain close liaison with the police and other law enforcement agencies and through taking over from the probation service much of the social enquiry work on juveniles. It is on the treatment side however that they will in future play their biggest role. The Act provides for a restricted range of treatment orders. Two of these are, respectively, the supervision order which replaces the probation order for the under-seventeens, and the care order which takes the place of the approved school order.

The new supervision order, while it retains much of the form of its predecessor, has two novel features. These are linked with what the White Paper called 'intermediate treatment', on the view which had often been expressed that some form of such treatment should be available to the courts which allows a youngster to remain living in his own home but which will bring him for a short time in contact with a different environment. This type of treatment was intended to be constructive, a positive aid to a youngster's social adjustment. The supervision order may be made for up to three years. In its first form intermediate treatment may stipulate residence for a period up to a maximum of ninety days in the first year of supervision. According to the White Paper this form of treatment is aimed at the children who have a really difficult home situation, where it is desirable to give them a 'breathing space' away from home and allow for some social work to be undertaken with their families. Coupled with this use or as an alternative to it, it can provide an opportunity for a youngster to obtain some short-term treatment in, for example, a local authority home or some other kind of residential establishment. In its second form, the order may involve short-term residence, attendance or participation for one or more periods of not more than thirty days during each year of supervision. The supervisor is free to decide on the kind of placement, depending on what he considers to be desirable in the youngster's interests, and will make his selection from whatever facilities are available. These could range over organized work projects, adventure training or social service. The intention is to allow the youngster to feel that he is doing something that is worth while and not that he is just 'doing time'. The care order becomes the modern version of the fit person order and incorporates the former approved school order. It will be used in the case of children and young persons who need to be removed from home for long spells of time. Similar to the powers which they had under the fit person order, the local authority will have freedom to place the youngster in whatever type of placement seems most suitable and is, of course, also available. Local authorities will have to provide a comprehensive range of residential facilities and the present range of establishments, such as reception centres, children's homes, remand homes, approved schools in future will be known by the generic title of 'community homes'. The approved school system, as a separate entity, will cease to exist. Some approved schools, about a quarter of the total in existence in 1968 were already being provided by local authorities and these will easily be incorporated under the new schemes. The remainder provided by various voluntary organizations have the option of coming into the new system. It will be open to the managers of any voluntary homes, including an approved school, to make their facilities available within the public system on a regular basis either as a community home, or as some may prefer, they may opt for inclusion in the state education system of residential establishments. There is, however, no legal obligation for voluntary homes to join either; they may decide to stay out altogether, in which case they still remain subject to registration and inspection and will be known as registered voluntary homes to distinguish them from those within the public system which will not need to be registered.

To give full effect to the provision of the wide range of facilities that will be required, local authorities' areas have been joined together to form twelve Joint Planning Committees. Their constituent membership will be appointed from children's committees or whoever their successors eventually will be and will also include representation from health and education committees. The work of these joint committees will be directly concerned with planning for the needs of a wide area, for instance Wales will be covered by one committee, and this will call for continuous study and appraisal of changing conditions.

The Act provides for the phasing in of the various procedures. A great deal of work is necessary to implement the administrative changes involved and it will also be some years before the necessary resources, including sufficient staff, will be available to enable the new procedures to be worked.

The changes embodied in the Act are not as abrupt as they may at first sight appear—just as Section 1 of the Children and Young Persons Act 1963 confirmed rather than initiated a trend that was already noticeable in the mid-fifties, so the provisions in the Act of 1969 similarly confirmed a trend. In recent years the problems of the young offender had increasingly been seen in the context of the problems of deprived children generally. It had become more realistic to seek the common factors between the delinquent, the emotionally disturbed, the maladjusted and other children who came to the notice of local authorities rather than stress the differences that might exist between them.

Naturally the administrative changes seem to mark off one period from another; as for example in the case of the approved school and the system of which it formed a part, but even there, in a few instances, notably in Oxfordshire, there had been a tendency for some years by the courts to prefer the fit person order to the approved school order leaving the local authority to secure something other than approved school treatment for the young offender. The all-embacing title of 'community home' also is but a convenient and suitably neutral one to describe the range of residential establishment which local authorities have built up, often carefully and after a great deal of thought, in their attempts to provide individualization of treatment. There are some innovations to be noted however—the new supervision order with its built-in treatment plans and of course the setting up of planning machinery to survey and plan across the existing local authority boundaries. These are constructive ideas which should yield some good results in the future.

Home Office reorganization

The change in the role of the child care service brings with it a change of central administration at the Home Office. The Central Training Council in Child Care was set up in 1947, and the Advisory Council in Child Care in 1948. The Children's Act also enlarged the functions of the inspectorate which had previously existed for some facets of the service. The inspectorate were expected to serve as the 'eyes and ears' of the Home Office, but the legislation said little of their precise functions. The essential purpose of inspection visits to local authorities was to ensure that Home Office regulations were being carried out. This is not to say that there was no more to the functions than that, but the focus on the more detailed aspects of statutory rules got in the way of concentrating on broader aspects of child care policy.[15] A wider role, however, is now officially encouraged. The child care inspector is seen as someone who can stimulate individual, group and community work, who has ideas about social needs and can inspire and help others to work them through.[16] No doubt the purely inspectorial role must remain but will form only a part of the inspector's functions in the future.

The Advisory Council and the Central Training Council have been reconstituted so as to become the central forum for the co-operative planning and discussion of research, development and training in child care. As part of this reconstitution, a new Development Group was formed in the Home Office Children's Department in 1968. It consists of members of Home Office staff, both administrative and professional. In its initial work it will concentrate on developments in residential care and, in particular, on the needs of those young people who under the former legislation were subject to approved school orders, so that the planning of community homes can take in the kind of provision that will be required to meet those needs. The Home Office research unit, which itself undertakes child care research projects, will be involved with assisting in the evaluation of new developments and of the new procedures and treatments.

All this implies a renewed spirit and a fresh urgency from the centre and although local authorities tend to be rather suspicious of Whitehall, many will welcome positive leadership and support. The quality of the child care service must in the final analysis depend on the quality of the people who are in direct contact with those for whose needs they cater and the key factor in this is the supply of trained social workers. This matter will be discussed in the next chapter.

Notes

1. 'Families With Problems', the Council for Children's Welfare and the Fisher Group, 1958.
2. D. Donnison, Peggy Jay, Mary Stewart, 'The Ingleby Report—

Three Critical Essays', Fabian Society, Research series 231, 1962, pp. 1-10.

3. 'Crime—A Challenge to Us All', Labour Party, 1964, pp. 13-20.

4. Cmnd. 2742, August 1965.

5. *Report of the Committee on Local Authority and Allied Personal Services* (Seebohm), Cmnd. 3703, 1968.

6. Quoted in *Child Care News*, edition No. 78, September 1968, p. 4.

7. B. J. Kahan, 'Child Care and a Social Service Department', *Social Work*, Vol. 25, No. 4, October 1968, p. 10.

8. *Royal Commission on Local Government in England* (Redcliffe-Maud), 1966-69, Cmnd. 4040, 1969.

9. Seebohm report, paras. 666-81.

10. *Hansard*, House of Lords, Vol. 298, No. 27, 29 January 1969, Cols. 1191-2.

11. Management of Local Government (Maud), Vol. 1, Report of the Committee, 1967.

12. See e.g. the resolutions adopted at the annual conference of the Association of Child Care Officers, 1969, quoted in *Child Care News*, edition No. 87, June 1969.

13. *Hansard*, House of Lords, Vol. 298, *op. cit.*, Cols. 1192-3.

14. Cmnd. 3601, April 1968.

15. For a brief account of the work of the inspectorate see J. A. G. Griffiths, *Central Departments and Local Authorities*, Allen & Unwin, 1965, pp. 371-81.

16. Cmnd. 3601. See also the advertisement for Children's Department inspectors in *Case Conferences*, Vol. 15, No. 7, November 1968, p. 297.

6

Manpower and training

Up to 1947 no recognized training existed for child care. Local authorities frequently employed health visitors to supervise foster children but in some cases they had a special children's officer who possessed a social science qualification. The Curtis Committee had been particularly insistent that specialized training should be provided both for residential and field staff. Their Interim Report had been concerned with training and led to the setting up of the Central Training Council in Child Care whose function was to be the organization of training courses. At the outset it was decided that field staff should be trained by universities while residential staff, because their courses would require to have a more practical bias, would train at non-university centres of education. This followed the Curtis recommendations.

Professional training commenced at four universities in 1947, briefly expanding to six before falling back again to four in 1950 as the early demand for places fell away. Initially courses were for 'boarding-out officers', the title 'child care course' was not adopted until 1954. Local authorities, to begin with, were slow to absorb professionally trained staff. It is probable, as the Younghusband Committee suggested in their report, that local authorities which had been making efforts for some years to recruit candidates with social science qualifications into their services, failed to differentiate between those courses and professional social work courses, assuming them to have equal value as preparations for social work.[1] As late as 1951 it was not unusual for a university-trained child care officer to have to wait months before finding a job. Expansion of training was also slow in the early fifties and did not really gather speed until the early sixties.

Many more women than men took up training. Up to the end of 1960, 681 women and 67 men had successfully completed their courses but even this moderate number did not appear to stay long in child care work. There was a disturbingly high wastage rate of staff, trained as well as untrained, and a low proportion of trained staff to untrained. In 1957 the Association of Children's Officers conducted a survey of staffing in children's departments.[2] It emerged that out of an establishment of 1,037 child care officers only about 25% were professionally fully qualified, although there were another 41% who had a social science qualification. An equally disquieting discovery was the quick turnover of staff. Of the establishment in 1957, 698 candidates had been appointed in the three years between 1954 and 1957 and the wastage due to resignations ran at the rate of about 47% of total establishment during the same period. In fact, what the Home Office itself referred to in 1961 as 'a grave shortage of trained staff' has continued virtually unabated to the present day, although it is now in part due to the very rapid expansion in staff establishment with which the training programme has not managed to keep pace.

Expansion of the service and the need to attract more people to enter training forced the Central Training Council to look outside the universities for courses. This opened up opportunities for mature and suitable non-graduates to take up training.

The Younghusband working party in 1959 had recommended training in colleges of commerce for people who wished to enter local authority health and welfare work, and the courses for the Certificate in Social Work established as a result of this recommendation provided the model for child care training courses. The first of these courses was established at the London North-West Polytechnic in 1960; since then similar courses have been established in other colleges and extra-mural departments of universities throughout the country. The assimilation of child care courses with courses for the Certificate in Social Work which have a very similar educational content, is under active consideration at the time of writing.

The training of residential workers was of equal importance to the training of field staff. Roughly a third of all the children in care each year between 1948 and 1960 were in various local authority residential homes, and they required a large number of people to look after them.

Local education authority colleges provided the bulk of training resources, but some voluntary organizations were able to help out with training since they already had a tradition of in-service training for their own staff. By the end of 1960, 1,772 women and 264 men had qualified for their Central Training Council Residential Care Certificate. However, the ratio of trained to untrained staff in residential care was even lower than that in fieldwork. Another survey sponsored by the Association of Children's Officers,[3] covering houseparents and assistant houseparents, revealed that of staff employed on 1 January 1958 only 239, or 9% of the 2,778 staff, held the Home

Office certificate, and 162 (6%) had some other relevant qualification. Turnover among residential staff was high, 28% for houseparents and 51% for assistant houseparents in 1957, the great majority leaving for reasons other than transfer within the service or retirement.

Staffing during the first twelve years or so of the service presented a succession of difficulties. The initial decision to recruit field staff trainees from university graduates or the equivalent, and to confine professional training to the universities meant that progress was bound to be slow. 'The courses are not always full, and many more applications would be welcomed ... from men and women with suitable education background and good experience', said the Home Office Children's Department Report of 1959. Publicity about the work and training opportunities was probably inadequate. As figures already quoted for the ratio of men to women taking training indicate, the child care service did not prove attractive to men, and the large intake of women produced a high staff turnover.

On the residential side, the rigours of the work coupled with the low salaries offered to houseparents and assistants limited recruitment from the start. In a period of full employment residential work had to offer something better than the many forms of alternative jobs available to women, and this it did not do.

Thus a manpower problem developed when the child care service was set up, particularly when the need for trained staff became more widely recognized. There were two problems: getting sufficient staff to man the service, and providing training. As functions expanded, especially after 1963, local authorities required more and more staff, particularly on the field side of the work. The first survey on staffing which was conducted by the Association of

Children's Officers in 1957, showed that there were a little over 1,000 established field officers' posts. Two follow-up surveys indicated that this number had gone up to 1,567 in 1962 and 1,980 in 1964. It was not possible to fill all these posts. In 1962 the proportion of vacancies to established posts was just under 8% and it rose to more than 12% in 1964.[4] In 1966 the total child care officer establishment was 2,675 and the Home Office forecast that about 3,800 posts would be required by 1970.[5] At that time, the new demands for staff consequent on the Children and Young Persons Act 1969 were not yet envisaged.

The local authority returns to the Home Office for 31 March 1969 indicated that there were 3,082 full-time field officers and 140 whole-time equivalent of part-time field officers in posts, together with 368 trainees in England and Wales. The wastage rate was 15·8% of officers in posts on 31 March 1968.

The supply of fully professionally trained staff lagged behind demand. The professional associations of children's officers and child care officers continually pressed for more trained staff and gradually too local authorities came to demand them; though there is a suspicion, if not concrete evidence, that some committee members still had to be discouraged from the view that child care could be undertaken by anyone with an abundance of good will and a tough physique.

Training facilities remained underdeveloped up to 1960. Only fifty students completed training in that year. After that date the position began to improve and the training programme gathered impetus each year as more and more training courses were opened, in the main at colleges of further education. In 1963, 171 candidates completed their training, in 1966, 242 and in 1968 more than 700 entered courses. An important development was the establishment in 1967 of a large emergency training course in London with an annual intake of 100 students. Since then a similar course has been scheduled to be located at Leeds.

Training brings its own problems; competent fieldwork supervisors were in short supply, and this hampered the expansion of courses or the setting-up of new ones. The solution to this problem will take time, for new supervisors have to be trained for the task and new ways of using existing supervisors have to be devised.

One encouraging aspect of the training situation was that more men were coming forward as candidates. As courses for mature students without formal university entrance qualifications got under way, the balance which formerly had been in favour of women was gradually being redressed. In 1966, of the 393 students entering training, 155 were men and 241 were women; in 1968 the figures were already coming much closer to each other—of 705 students entering courses, 303 were men and 402 women.

The importance of this development lay in the stabilization of the employment situation. For many years the service had been losing trained young women who left work after a few years to marry and start families. Lack of staff continuity is bad for clients and the service alike. Clients never get a chance to get used to one worker, and the service never gets the opportunity of benefiting from the experience of the young, newly trained worker. Further, rapid staff turnover is extremely wasteful and expensive.

As training facilities have increased, the proportion of fully professionally trained staff to total field staff has gradually risen. In 1962 it was 26%, in 1969 it had gone up to 38·5% and if we include those officers who have other acceptable professional social work qualifications, the proportion was 42·2%.

Distribution of fully trained staff however continued to be uneven. In 1969, the London boroughs were comparatively well off with 45·9%, next came the county councils with 41·9% and last came the county boroughs with 28·8%. Even this can only give a very generalized picture. The Association of Children's Officers survey for 1964 for instance showed that while a few local authorities had as high a proportion as 90% of trained staff, others, at that time had none at all.

The position of trained and qualified staff for residential work had improved only marginally in the sixties compared with the fifties. The A.C.O. survey indicated that in 1964 only 10¼% of residential staff (apart from staff in residential nurseries where the position was better) had the Home Office Letter of Recognition in Residential Child Care, while a further 7½% had some other relevant qualification. The high wastage rates which were discovered in the earlier surveys were continuing, the situation with regard to residential staff being as serious as that for field staff. Miss Sylvia Watson commented in 1964, 'If wastage rate is estimated as the ratio of vacancies occurring during the year to the total number of established posts, the wastage rates for child care officers and children's home staff are both 28% while for residential nurseries, which employ a higher proportion of young women, the wastage rate is 42%'.[6] In actual numbers this meant that not far short of 1,500 people left the residential service in any one year. In 1966 it was estimated that there were a total of 5,600 staff, 84% of whom were in full-time posts.[7]

A report on residential staffing needs was published in 1967. This was the Williams report,[8] the result of a privately sponsored enquiry which dealt, amongst other relevant matters, with training. The committee recommended a common two-year training with specialist options, for all newcomers to residential work. Potential residential child care staff would therefore train with others who intend to make a career in different residential services, for instance in old people's homes or in homes for mentally handicapped adults. This idea for common training makes sense but doubt has been expressed in some quarters whether a two year course is a realistic proposition for the near future, bearing in mind the great needs for at least minimally trained staff in all the residential social work services including child care. The Williams Committee made no analysis of the actual work undertaken by different staff to justify a two-year training. It may be that varying skills are required for different types of work. In the short run, the argument runs, a compromise between quality and quantity may not be unreasonable.

Despite the urgent demand for basic training which absorbed the major part of the limited resources available, it became possible to set up advanced courses. This had become vital if residential work was to make any progress. The advanced courses quite clearly were intended to provide the stimulus for deeper study and new thinking. In 1968 there were two such courses and twelve others which provided the basic training. Between them they took 330 students.

A small-scale beginning was also made in providing a joint training for field and residential staff, something that was obviously well worth experimenting with despite the fact that the joint training process raised special problems.

During the sixties the need for fully trained, professionally qualified staff gained fuller acceptance and a greater sense of urgency was being demonstrated by the Home Office; but it still proved difficult to keep pace. Local authorities constantly needed additional staff, and since trained workers were in short supply they had perforce to take on untrained ones. This led some authorities to develop their own in-service training programmes for new recruits whom they could at a later stage second to training courses.

Training also had to be devised both by the Central Training Council and the local authorities to help equip staff for the senior jobs at middle management level, e.g. area officers and staff and student supervisors. With the growth of children's departments, an elaborate staff hierarchy evolved and this meant that more senior staff had to receive some form of training for their new positions. This new task, added to the tasks of training new entrants and untrained staff in post, has thrown a great strain on the available resources, and set up problems which to date are still far from solution.

Notes

1. *Report of the Working Party on Social Workers in the Local Authority Health and Welfare Services* (Younghusband), H.M.S.O., 1959, para. 819.

2. A.C.O. Bulletin, No. 65, August 1957.

3. A.C.O. Bulletin No. 78, September 1958.

4. S. Watson, 'Manpower in the Child Care Service', *Social Work*, Vol. 21, No. 1, January 1964, pp. 15-20, and a further note in *Social Work*, Vol. 21, No. 3, July 1964, pp. 31-2.

5. Home Office Report 1964-66, *op. cit.*, ch. III.
6. S. Watson, *op. cit.*
7. Seebohm report, *op. cit.*, Appx. F., para. 51.
8. National Council of Social Service, *Caring for People* (Williams Report), Allen & Unwin, 1967.

7
Postscript

Even a brief account of developments over twenty-two years in the child care service cannot be left without comment by way of conclusion. Some comparisons can be made between child care in 1948 and 1970 and some expectations as well as fears must be voiced about the future of the service.

In 1948 child care was a comparatively minor social service, created specifically for a group of children loosely designated as being 'deprived'. In practice it referred for the most part to those who had perforce to leave home because of some family misfortune. The work was concentrated on the care aspect, departments concerning themselves with the child in their care, away from his home, ensuring that his physical, mental and especially his emotional needs were met as well as available facilities allowed. This was a natural reaction to the deficiencies uncovered by the Curtis Committee. There was an emphasis on fostering because it was considered that, adoption apart, the foster home was likely to provide the best substitute to natural, family life; and when the supply of foster homes proved short of demand, the so-called family group homes were developed. Early rehabilitation with the family was the objective, and the period in care was intended to be as short as possible; but rehabilitation proved as difficult in practice as finding sufficient suitable foster homes. The numbers in care rose, straining the departments' resources to the limit.

Children's departments were already getting their quota of young offenders through committals to care by the courts, and the departments shared in care or protection work and approved school after-care functions. Once in care, distinctions between delinquents and non-delinquents did not apply; but most delinquent children remained outside the scope of the service.

In its early years then, the service was mainly a curative one, busy with the child in care or about to come into care.

It was some time before child care could establish its claim to available resources against those of other powerful local authority departments, in particular health and education. Both of these departments formerly had a share in the work of caring for deprived children; the scope of their operations still overlapped with those of the Children's Department to some extent; and both were inclined to look on the newcomer with something less than goodwill. Children's committees were the newest of the statutory local authority committees and possessed less prestige than the older ones. At the outset there was often a considerable turnover on children's committees as members gained sufficient seniority and party standing to move over to some more sought-after committee.[1]

The number of cases dealt with increased rapidly year by year. It is difficult to say whether this was because of a backlog of undiscovered need, or because the service became known as approachable and sympathetic. The pressure of cases and the interest shown in maternal deprivation theory made children's departments first look at the possibilities of preventive action. 'Would it not be preferable to provide a fence at the top of the cliff rather than an ambulance at the foot?' was a metaphor which found currency in the early fifties. And with the growth in numbers came additional duties leading departments to pay attention more and more to functions on the perimeter of the purely in-care functions.

Today the service is still growing. Its practitioners and commentators have been active in making it known to the general public, and it is frequently featured in official quarters and in the press. It has also developed a considerable literature of its own, always a sign of the extent of interest shown in a field of activity.

The skills of child care have become more refined, although these have developed more in the direction of diagnosis—as witnessed by the extensive use of case conferences—than treatment. The service now concerns itself not only with the needs of the child in care, though this is still the primary task, but more and more with the delinquent child outside care, with adoption, with the child caught up in his parents' matrimonial disputes, and, through preventive work, more broadly with the family and a multiplicity of problems not necessarily directly involving the care of children. The Children and Young Persons Act 1969 will widen the scope still further.

The service has become more highly professionalized. The influx of trained staff has influenced standards of work. Trained staff have insisted on being given the facilities for making the best use of their skills, and departments have been able to develop in-service training.

In Chapter 2 it was suggested that welfare work for children is not the monopoly of the child care service but that other services share in it on a broad front. The lines which demarcate functions are blurred and there is much overlap of services. The Seebohm Committee had a good deal to say about this and its recommendations centred in part around the need for eliminating these boundaries. Even if the Seebohm recommendations were to be fully implemented, there would necessarily still remain boundary areas where child care functions shade into education or health functions just as they have done ever since the new service was carried out; but, as suggested earlier, personal social service reorganization along Seebohm lines might lead to the submergence of the child care service. We would then have to ask: 'Where does *social work* begin and education end?', rather than 'Where does *child care* begin and education end?'

Finally, in this brief chapter one must pose the question whether child care is not really providing a patching-up service, dealing largely with symptoms of social problems rather than tackling causes. How far is poor housing responsible for children being received into care? Would the changes in public attitudes towards unmarried mothers help to reduce the steady flow of illegitimate children into care? Would the large number of children who come into care each year on account of their mothers' short-term illnesses or confinements be reduced if the home-help and day nursery services were to be substantially improved? Could not much more be done to provide special schools for maladjusted children and thus reduce the burden which the shortage of such school places imposes on children's departments?[2] Would better family allowances not go a long way to easing the problems associated with preventive work?

These are questions which raise fundamental issues of

social policy, social planning and the distribution of resources but they should continue to be asked, not least
by the practitioners themselves.

It must be conceded that to a large extent the child
care service fulfils a patching-up function. But one need
make no apology for this, for until the causes of deprivation and family breakdown can be uncovered, and
remedied or alternative services built up in sufficient
strength, people still need to be helped. Many of the problems the service deals with involve complex issues of
human relations which demand attention here and now.
It is in answering such urgent calls for help that the child
care service has built up a reputation during the past two
decades.

Notes

1. For an interesting critique of the part played by the com-
mittee system in the child care service in its early years, see G. M.
Kammerer, *British and American Child Welfare Services*, Wayne
State U.P., 1962, pp. 129-46.

2. In a recent survey undertaken by Lancashire County Council,
it was found that of 118 disturbed children in care of the county,
13 attended residential schools for the maladjusted but only 3 of
them could receive schooling within the geographic county; 8
of the remaining 10 had to travel over 100 miles to receive suitable education. See T. White in *Community Homes and the
Approved School System, op. cit.*

Guide to further reading

The literature on the child care service has built up to quite extensive proportions over the past two decades. Below are listed some of the publications which will prove valuable to the student who wishes to extend his knowledge of the subject.

Introductory and Historical:

J. PARFIT (editor), *The Community's Children*, Longmans. Contains a series of articles by various specialists in the child care field aimed at the general reader.

P. BOSS, 'Child Care and the Development of a Family Service', in Penelope Hall's *Social Services of England and Wales*, editor A. Forder, Routledge & Kegan Paul. A brief introduction to child care and future trends.

J. BOWLBY, *Child Care and the Growth of Love*, Pelican. This is a revised version of the original monograph, written to reach the wider public.

J. HEYWOOD, *Children in Care*, second edition, Routledge & Kegan Paul. A well-known, historical study of the subject.

E. PUGH, *Social Work in Child Care*, Routledge & Kegan Paul. A descriptive account of the various functions of the child care service.

J. STROUD, *The Shorn Lamb*, Longmans. Written as a novel it presents an amusing, yet penetrating account of the early years of the child care service.

J. STROUD, *An Introduction to the Child Care Service*, Longmans. Provides good coverage of the subject although it stops short of events over the past five years, but is still worthwhile reading.

A. F. YOUNG & E. T. ASHTON, *British Social Work in the Nineteenth Century*, Routledge & Kegan Paul. Contains a good summary of the Poor Law and voluntary organizations' work in relation to children in former years.

Special Aspects and Research Studies:

R. BALBERNIE, *Residential Work With Children*, Pergamon. This is an advanced study of residential work and takes an analytical approach.

T. FERGUSON, *Children in Care—and after*, Oxford University Press. A study of a group of Glasgow children who came into the care of the local authority.

I. GOODACRE, *Adoption Policy and Practice*, Allen & Unwin. This is a critical enquiry into current adoption practices and the assumptions on which these practices are based. The study was limited to the administrative area of one children's department.

J. A. G. GRIFFITHS, *Central Departments and Local Authorities*, Allen & Unwin. Analyses the relationship between Whitehall and local authorities in respect of a number of social services including child care which is dealt with in Chapter 6. There is a particularly valuable discussion in this chapter on the role of the Home Office inspectorate, a topic about which little had been written previously.

M. L. KELLMER PRINGLE (editor), *Caring for Children*, Longmans. This is a symposium on Co-operation in Child Care —it includes contributions on concepts of child care, co-operation principles and practice in relation to special groups of children and parents.

J. PACKMAN, *Child Care: Needs and Numbers*, Allen & Unwin. A comprehensive survey of the conditions which result in a child being received into care, it points to the differences in policies and practices between children's departments.

R. A. PARKER, *Decision in Child Care*, Allen & Unwin. A research study of a group of foster children analysing in particular factors which make for success or failure in fostering.

G. TRASLER, *In Place of Parents*, Routledge & Kegan Paul. This is an early research study, which preceded Dr Parker's and similarly focused on the outcome of fostering of a group of children.

D. LAMBERT (editor), *Residential Staff in Child Care*. Annual Review of the Residential Child Care Association, 1968. Contains sections dealing with topics of management principles and practices, internal dynamics and student supervision in the residential child care setting.

Summaries of research studies have been published under the auspices of the National Bureau for Co-operation in Child Care in association with Longmans. The relevant titles are:

R. DINNAGE & M. L. KELLMER PRINGLE, *Residential Child Care—Facts and Fallacies* and *Foster Home Care—Facts and Fallacies.*

M. L. KELLMER PRINGLE, *Adoption—Facts and Fallacies.*

Official Publications:

Report of the Care of Children Committee, 1946; Cmnd. 6922 (Curtis Report).

Report of the Committee on Children and Young Persons 1960; Cmnd. 1191 (Ingleby Report).

Report of the Committee on Children and Young Parents (Scotland), 1964; Cmnd. 2306 (Kilbrandon Report).

The Child, the Family and the Young Offender, 1965; Cmnd. 2742.

Children in Trouble, 1968; Cmnd. 3601.

Report of the Committee on Local Authority and Allied Personal Social Services, 1968; Cmnd. 3703 (Seebohm Report).

The Home Office periodically publishes an account on the work of its children's department. At the time of writing the most recent report covers the period 1964-66. It is available through H.M.S.O.